THE COMPLETE IDIOT'S GUIDE® TO

Walking for Health

by Erika Peters

alpha books

A Pearson Education Company

International Standard Book Number: 0-02-864002-0
Library of Congress Catalog Card Number: Available upon request.

03   02   01   8   7   6   5   4   3   2

Interpretation of the printing code: The rightmost number of the first series of numbers is the year of the book's printing; the rightmost number of the second series of numbers is the number of the book's printing. For example, a printing code of 01-1 shows that the first printing occurred in 2001.

Printed in the United States of America

Publisher
Marie Butler-Knight

Product Manager
Phil Kitchel

Managing Editor
Jennifer Chisholm

Senior Acquisitions Editor
Randy Ladenheim-Gil

Development Editor
Suzanne LeVert

Senior Production Editor
Christy Wagner

Copy Editor
Jan Zunkel

Illustrator
Jody Schaeffer

Cover Designers
Mike Freeland
Kevin Spear

Book Designers
Scott Cook and Amy Adams of DesignLab

Indexer
Brad Herriman

Layout/Proofreading
Angela Calvert
John Etchison
Mary Hunt
Gloria Schurick

Contents at a Glance

Contents

Foreword

Whenever I recommend fitness walking to people, they often respond with an expression of disbelief and curiosity. They ask, "Can walking really help me get fit?" The expression and question come from years of conditioning that has taught us that exercise isn't effective unless it's uncomfortable or painful. But as fitness trainer Erika Peters knows, one of the best things you can do for your health is unlearn the "no pain, no gain" myth. Erika wants people to know that exercise doesn't have to be a white-knuckle, kamikaze endurance mission to be effective. That's one of the reasons she wrote this book.

The Complete Idiot's Guide to Walking for Health corroborates what I and a handful of other forward-thinking fitness experts have been saying for some time: You don't have to work out for hours and hours to get fit, and you don't have to obsess over your diet. With the right exercise program you can look great, feel great, and still have a normal, balanced life.

Whether you're just starting to walk for fitness or if you like the challenge of trekking steep inclines while wearing a weighted vest, walking can offer a lifetime of increasingly challenging workouts. And if you're of a mind to venture beyond, walking can be a gateway to other kinds of activities, such as cycling or running. Can walking help you get fit? You bet it can. The beauty of fitness walking is there are no prerequisites. You can start from where you are right now.

That brings us to the question, what does "fitness" mean to you? Does it mean a certain dress size? Does it mean getting rid of your love handles? Better aerobic conditioning? More shapely legs? More vitality? Whatever your goals, there are undoubtedly a number of ways to achieve them and even more ways to waste time and energy by taking the wrong approach. In other words, you need a specific plan that will take you directly to your goals with no detours. As a professional trainer who has taught hundreds of thousands of people about various aspects of fitness through my workshops, writing, and coaching, I'm convinced that this book provides such a plan.

The Complete Idiot's Guide to Walking for Health will teach you, step by step, everything you need to know about walking for health. But it doesn't stop there: You'll learn how to measure your progress, how to make walking a habit, and how to turn up the heat after you've mastered the basics. You'll learn about nutrition, weight loss, strength training, and concerns for special populations, such as people who live with diabetes or hypertension. In short, you'll learn a great deal about your body and your mind. Written in simple language, this book will motivate you to take immediate action.

Read on, because you're in for a treat. Erika is passionate about her work, and I'm confident that her love for fitness and her concern for you will shine through on the pages that follow. Remember, Erika's not just a writer—she's a trainer. And this book is for you.

If you haven't figured it out yet, you're very close to achieving your fitness goals. I teach my own students that the shortest distance between their existing physical condition and total fitness is a straight line, and I encourage them to do what works to find their own, personal straight line. Let me be the first to congratulate you for finding yours.

Alex Singleton
President of Metamorphosis Personal Training, Founder of Fitness University

Introduction

"A journey of a thousand miles begins with a single step."

—Confucius

What could be easier than walking? Efficient, accessible, and easy to do, walking is one of the best modes of exercise today. All you need is a good pair of shoes and you are on your way. Walking is rapidly becoming one of the most favorite forms of physical activity because it can be done anywhere, at any time, and by anyone. Plus, it's cheap!

How to Use This Book

In **Part 1, "Building a Daily Habit for Health's Sake,"** I explain some of the many ways that walking improves both your physical and your mental health. I show you how to determine your level of fitness now, as well as where you can take it in the future. This is the part of the book where you learn what it means to commit to health, both now and for many years to come.

In **Part 2, "Progressing Safely,"** I introduce you to ways that you can make your walking routine more challenging. I also provide some suggestions on how to spice up your workouts to prevent boredom. In addition, I explain why strength training and flexibility are important components to a complete fitness routine, and I include some sample exercises you can do whether you are just beginning or have been at it for a while. Finally, I show you how to tell if you're overtaxing your system, in addition to explaining why it's important to schedule days off and take breaks when needed.

As you move on to **Part 3, "Walking for Weight Loss,"** you'll learn about issues related to weight (both loss and maintenance of) and how to break away from poor habits. Here you'll explore reasons why being overweight can be a hazard to your health and possible reasons why it has become a problem for you. You will learn how to make healthier choices for the future, and how walking can get your weight and your life back on track.

Part 4, "Walking as a Lifestyle," is a cool part because I get to explain fun ways you can incorporate more walking into your daily doings. Be it walking to work or walking vacations, you will learn tips on changing your routine and your attitude toward exercise. Finally, we look at ways to avoid excuses, as well as learn some tricks that will help keep you motivated when the going gets tough.

In **Part 5, "Your Feet,"** I introduce various common injuries associated with walking. I explain how you can treat them, as well as ways to avoid them in the future. You'll learn about the difference between orthopedists and podiatrists, and get some guidelines on how to choose the proper footwear to keep your feet happy, healthy, and injury-free.

In addition to the text of the chapters, you'll see many pieces of "extra" information in sidebars scattered throughout the chapters. I have grouped these into four distinct types, each with a sports-game theme:

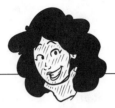

Interesting Excerpts

Facts, statistics, interesting quotations and information meant to notify, inspire, and motivate the reader.

Walkers Watch Out!

These are warnings and precautions meant to alert the reader to pay attention to high-risk moves and or unhealthy attitudes.

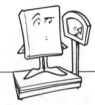

Weighty Words

These are terms and definitions that the reader may find useful as he or she incorporates healthy habits and activities into daily life.

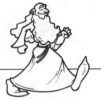

Wise Walkers

These are tips, suggestions, and other positive ideas for the reader to use as he or she begins to design or modify their approach to exercise.

In summary, I would like you to look at this book as a reference tool; something you can use whenever you need it. Simply explained and easy to read, *The Complete Idiot's Guide to Walking for Health* will provide you with a wealth of information that you can use now, as well as many years down the road.

"Let him that would move the world, first move himself."

—Socrates

Acknowledgments

My first thanks goes to Andree Abecassis, my literary agent, who sought me out to write this book. Without her encouragement, this book would not have been possible, and I thank her tremendously for opening this new world to me and for helping me to believe that anything can be done "one step at a time." I also want to express gratitude to the staff at Pearson Education and in particular Randy Ladenheim-Gil, Suzanne LeVert, Christy Wagner, and Jan Zunkel for being clear, concise, but most of all encouraging, despite all of my questions and confusion.

Thanks to my 93-year-old grandma, who, to this day, continues to take her weekly walks around the block and who gives me inspiration as I look forward to my later years. I am also deeply indebted to my parents who taught me the value of family, good health, and an active lifestyle from day one. Much gratitude to my brother Nick and my sister Christiane for offering me their support and their love, as well as free reign over the computer for months, no questions asked. Also, a giant thanks to my sister Sabrina who helped me with the photo sessions and who, despite the lack of good lighting, did a phenomenal job. And finally a huge hug to my boyfriend, Ariel, who always says the right thing at the right time and who continues to support me and encourage me to be the best that I can be.

Trademarks

All terms mentioned in this book that are known to be or are suspected of being trademarks or service marks have been appropriately capitalized. Alpha Books and Pearson Education cannot attest to the accuracy of this information. Use of a term in this book should not be regarded as affecting the validity of any trademark or service mark.

Part 1

Building a Daily Habit for Health's Sake

It's so easy to find excuses not to exercise. You're too busy at work, you've got to drive the kids to and from soccer practice, and you've got to go grocery shopping and cook dinner. With all of these responsibilities, how on earth can anyone find time for something so luxurious as a walk around the block?

Walking may be considered a luxury, but it's really a necessity if you want to stay healthy. I know that you've got all these errands and "to do" lists to complete, but without your health, you might not have the wherewithal to do any activities. In this part of the book, I'll explain how exercise, and walking in particular, can be beneficial to your health. You'll go through a series of fitness evaluations that will determine your starting point. I'll also show you ways to find time and commit to a walking program, in addition to suggesting good gear to get you going.

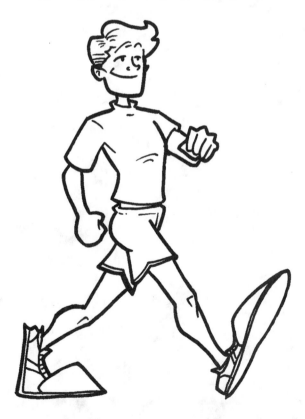

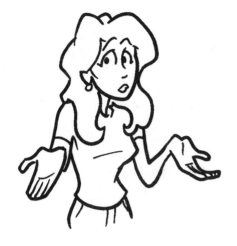

Chapter 1

Why Walk?

In This Chapter

➤ The mental benefits of walking

➤ Why walking is good for your health

➤ The positive effects of walking on your soul

➤ The easiest exercise around

Why walk? Perhaps the real question we should ask ourselves is "Why not walk?" Walking is not only one of the more efficient and inexpensive forms of exercise around, it also offers an array of psychological, physical, and spiritual benefits as well. That's right—an exercise that works on you from head to toe as well as from the inside out.

In this chapter, I'll show you how you can, by the simple act of putting one foot in front of the other, reduce stress, decrease your risk of a heart attack, increase your creative and occupational capacity—and that's just a brief list of potential benefits.

The Importance of Walking

With the introduction of technology and computers, it seems that our society is becoming more and more sedentary. The hours we all spend in cars, in planes, and sitting at our desks at work have increased more in the last two decades than in the 10 decades before them. The Internet has provided access to almost everything from books to broccoli, making taking a walk to the local bookstore or grocery store a burden and a "waste of time." With the simple click of a few buttons, you can have anything you need without having to leave your house or even your chair!

Unfortunately, all of this sitting is not good for you. Beyond the fact that your buttocks are getting flatter (and fatter), sitting for long periods of time distorts your natural muscle balance, decreases your energy, and stiffens your joints. It's no wonder so many of us have chronic pain!

The good news is you don't have to develop all these problems. The bad news is there is no magic potion or special recipe that will whip you into shape effortlessly. You have to work at it, at least a bit. All you really have to do is move more, get up and walk around, to get your blood flowing and your muscles growing. Walking is a perfect means to achieve both goals. Cheap, available, and easy (mind out of the gutter please), walking offers you most everything you need for a happier and healthier life. We'll start with the benefits that walking on a regular basis will have on your mental health.

Mental Health Motivators

Depression is no longer a "closet" term. Many Americans suffer some form of depression from mild mood disorders to far more serious bouts, and they are speaking out about it. Anti-depressants such as Zoloft and Prozac are being prescribed in record amounts. Drug and alcohol abuse is on the rise as people turn to "quick fixes" to deal with their stress and depression. We are a nation in crisis, yet it seems that no one knows how to deal with it.

Anxiety, stress, and panic disorders are other mental illnesses that are increasing in number as we become busier and busier. Our bodies have become so used to feeling constant fatigue and tension that we hardly even notice it anymore. Without adequate exercise, sleep, and a healthy diet, however, this stress can easily turn into a host of mental and emotional problems, including (but not limited to) insomnia, weight gain, and panic attacks.

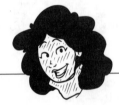

Interesting Excerpts

Stress is the disease of the modern age. It is an early warning sign telling us that we are not in control of our lives and that we need to take action. Stress has many causes, but most experts agree that lack of exercise is a major factor. We need to become more active—and the easiest and safest way is to begin a fitness walking program.

—From *The Rhythm for Life—Seven Highly Effective Ways to Walk Away from Stress,* by Les Snowdon

Although it has not been proven, many experts agree that our busy lives have contributed to the rise of psychological problems and other mental health disorders. In fact, the American Institute of Stress claims that stress has been linked to all the leading causes of death, including heart disease, cancer, lung ailments, accidents, cirrhosis, and suicide. The Institute cites a three-year study conducted by a large corporation that showed that 60 percent of employee absences were due to psychological problems such as stress.

Perhaps it's the disconnection from other people that leaves us feeling isolated and blue. Maybe it's the lack of free time for creativity and spontaneity. Or perhaps it's the pressure to succeed and to keep up with everyone else. Whatever the reason, this stress is bad and getting worse, and it is something we must start paying attention to.

So how in the world can walking help? Well, for starters, exercise produces chemicals in your body known as *endorphins*. Endorphins serve as your body's natural painkillers and are released into your system when your body is under a certain amount of physical stress (from exercise). Ever heard anyone refer to getting a "natural high" during or after his or her workout? They probably feel that way thanks to the endorphin released in their bloodstream. Endorphins are all natural, free, and good for you— chemicals that make you feel euphoric when you exercise. A shot of the endorphin rush two to four times a week might be just what you need to elevate your blue moods.

People who feel down can literally walk the blues away. Not only does exercise help distract you from your negative thoughts, it also forces you to go outside into the world, to realize that there is a world out there, not just the dark little one you've been trapped in. It makes you feel good, which promotes positive thoughts. You are doing something healthy for yourself, and it feels right. All you have to do is take that first step.

What I'm getting at here is that walking creates a sense of self-confidence and overall well-being. Getting out and doing something good for your body is invigorating and inspirational. Walking also serves as a healthy social outlet. Having little time for friends, significant others, and/or children is another negative side effect of our busy lives. We start to feel cut off and isolated from those important to us. Being alone a lot can nourish negative thought

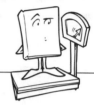

Weighty Words

Endorphins (abbreviation for endogenous morphine) are a special class of opiate-like substances released by the brain's pituitary gland. They produce feelings of euphoria and block the sensation of pain.

Wise Walkers

Perhaps the hardest time to motivate yourself to exercise is when you are feeling down. This is also the most important time. Force yourself if you must. Don't think too much. Just get out there.

Wise Walkers

Going for a walk with the kids after dinner or taking the pup for a stroll are other ways to spend some quality time with those important to you.

Walkers Watch Out!

Even though exercise is said to decrease certain incidents of depression and anxiety, not everyone can solve their mental problems so easily. Consult your physician or local counseling center for more information if your mood is interfering with your daily life.

patterns and feelings of isolation. By taking up walking with a friend, you'll not only get in shape but you'll also catch up on lost time.

I'm not asking for much here. All you need is a quick 30-minute walk three to five times a week to decrease your stress and anxiety levels. That's it! Of course, if you'd like to do more, go right ahead. The point is, walking enables you to take a step away (literally) from your hectic life. It gives you a little break to stand up so you can settle down. It also helps reduce muscle tension and stiff joints caused by being so still for prolonged periods of time. Getting the blood and oxygen flowing to the muscles and brain increases brain activity and clarity of mind, and it promotes an overall sense of well-being.

A Walking Body Is a Healthy Body

So, walking helps mend your mind. Now, what other benefits can you get from a joyful jaunt, you ask? Improved health, for starters. Consider the fact that millions of Americans suffer from heart attacks annually. In fact, according to the American Heart Association, coronary heart disease is America's number-one killer.

Even though it may appear that every Tom, Dick, and Harry (or Sue, Lynn, and Mary) is on a diet, the unfortunate fact is, we are getting larger and larger by the moment. Weight-related diseases such as diabetes and high blood pressure are on the rise. One would think that, with all of the information and education on health and disease available, we'd all be fit as fiddles. But we're not.

Indeed, we are a tremendously sedentary population. We don't grow up thinking of walking as an option, no matter how short the distance. Certain newer cities are even sidewalk-less, leaving you no choice but to drive. And we like to drive. We are a car-loving nation. Drive-through fast food, money machines, and dry-cleaning are just a few of the activities we can perform without having to leave our seat behind the wheel.

A Heart-to-Heart About Your Heart

A heart attack results from too little oxygen getting to the heart. Our arteries become clogged from high cholesterol (poor diets), smoking, inactivity, and high blood pressure. The vessels carrying blood to and from the heart harden and narrow causing a condition known as *atherosclerosis*. As a result, the heart has to work harder to deliver the blood we need to our working muscles. Eventually, our hearts get tired and weaken from all of this hard work, resulting in heart failure.

Thank goodness there is help. With a regular walking routine, you can decrease your risk of such a morbid fate. As you move more, you will start to feel better. When you feel better you want to eat better, which eventually lowers weight and cholesterol levels. Lower cholesterol means cleaner arteries. As our arteries clear, our blood pressure drops, putting less pressure on the heart. This, in turn, allows more oxygen-rich blood to be delivered throughout the body. With more oxygen and blood moving around, more waste products and other toxins are being eliminated from our system. Within months we are feeling more energetic and alive.

Beautiful, Bountiful Bones

Osteoporosis, or decreased bone density, is commonly associated with an older population, but younger people are at risk as well. When bones have not had any stress put on them (i.e., weight-bearing activity) they become dry and brittle, and they fracture and break easily. Because of our increasingly sedentary lifestyles, our bones are not receiving the necessary load they need to stay strong and durable.

Thankfully, your body has an amazing capacity for repair and, with just a few minor changes, can heal itself back to health. Walking three to five days a week at a moderate pace for 20 to 30 minutes, combined with two or three days of weight training, helps build strong, sturdy bones. It also helps build bone-supporting muscles, taking some of the pressure off your joints and decreasing your risk of injury.

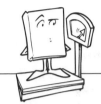

Weighty Words

Atherosclerosis literally means "hardening of the arteries." It is a disease that causes thickening and stiffness of the wall of the artery, leading to serious consequences. In fact, over one half of all deaths in the United States are a direct or indirect result of atherosclerosis, making it the single largest "killer disease" of them all.

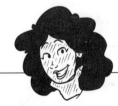

Interesting Excerpts

The American Heart Association now has a Web site called "Just Move," which contains information on heart disease and strokes as well as fitness facts and health issues. Take a look at www. justmove.com and learn more about your heart.

Weighty Issues

The number-one thing that comes out of most of my clients' mouths when we first discuss their goals is, "I want to lose this!" as they point accusingly at their mid-section. Losing weight usually is the fuel that ignites the fire and desire to exercise. And who can blame you? The media is filled with thin, pre-pubescent–type icons whose body-fat percentages give definition to the mathematical notion "decimal." The pressure to be thin is everywhere!

Although I do not embrace the message behind the saying "thin is in," I do believe that staying within a certain weight range will help you maintain your optimum health. Being overweight can cause any number of problems including diabetes, heart disease, and high blood pressure. Not to mention the fact that it can be extremely painful and uncomfortable on your joints.

Walking is one of the safest forms of exercise to help you lose and maintain your weight. Because it is primarily low impact (you always keep one foot on the ground during your workout), pressure on the joints is minimal. In addition, the level of workload can easily be adjusted. Too hard? All you have to do is slow down. Too easy? Find a hill and pick up the pace. Furthermore, it is uncomplicated and easy to do, requiring little coordination and skill. All you have to do is know how to tie your shoes and you are out the door!

Enticingly Energetic

Have you ever heard people describe the phenomenon of feeling more energy once they've started exercising? How can this be possible? One would think that more energy out (exercising) equals less energy in (yawn), right? Not quite. By exercising, you improve your body's ability to deliver blood and oxygen to your muscles. This then brings more nutrients (energy) to the working tissues. Here's how it works:

1. You step out your door and begin your walk.
2. Your muscles begin to work faster and harder, signaling to the heart and lungs that they need more fuel.
3. Your breath increases in depth and speed in an attempt to take in more air.
4. More oxygen fills the lungs and is filtered into the blood.
5. Oxygen-rich blood is then delivered to the heart.
6. The heart pumps faster to keep up with the rest of the body's need for blood.
7. More blood and oxygen are delivered to the working muscles.

Once everything is synchronized, the muscles respond by moving faster and with more ease. Over time, the lungs expect this added need for oxygen and they expand. The heart also responds happily by growing in size and strength so it can push more blood out to the body with fewer beats. With larger lungs and a bigger heart, more blood, nutrients, and oxygen are being delivered through your body on a more consistent basis, thus providing a steady stream of energy. This boosts muscle endurance and an overall greater capacity for everyday activities. Hence, the explanation for all those energetic exercisers you keep coming across.

Joint Adventures

Walking also helps build the strength and integrity of your joints. With greater blood flow, more oxygen and nutrients are being delivered to your bone structures. This not only helps to keep the bone supple and healthy, it also assists in carrying the waste products, associated with stiff joints, out of the bone structures themselves. With stronger bones come more tenacious connective tissues such as ligaments and tendons, tissues that help with the support and movement of your muscles and bones. When you take care of them with proper exercise and nutrition, they become stronger, helping you to avoid injury as well as everyday aches and pains.

Balancing Acts

Sitting at a desk, staring at a computer 12 inches from your face is hardly what I'd call a major physical challenge. Other than furiously tapping away at your keyboard, your body isn't moving a whole heck of a lot. With so little practice at using the skills your body was built to perform, you risk losing some of your most innate capabilities, such as depth perception and coordination. This, in turn, increases your chances of getting hurt and injured while performing even the most common of activities.

Walking helps with your balance. Sensory perception, foot-eye coordination, and muscle control are just some of the many things going on between our brains and our limbs on a second-to-second basis. However natural these functions may seem, they can diminish over time with age and underuse. That's why walking is a perfect way to keep in practice and to stay in shape at the same time.

Soulful Strides: Why Walking Is Good for the Soul

So now we've covered the mind and the body. What else is there? Let's see, mind, body and …. How about the soul? What does walking do for our peace of mind? Well, for one, it serves as a break from work, studying, and/or the kids. It also provides a little privacy and meditation to regain some perspective, inspiration, and creativity. Finally, it enables you to get in touch with nature. It gives you a sense of belonging to something larger than yourself, something magical and eternal.

Pausing for Breath

Ever hear the expression "all work and no play makes Jack a dull boy"? With so many things to do and so little time to do them, the first thing we often compromise is

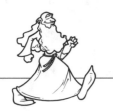

Wise Walkers

Instead of eating lunch at your desk tomorrow, try going for a 15- to 20-minute walk. This little "breather" will replenish the oxygen in your body, get your juices flowing, and ease your worrying mind for a few moments. It also helps to break up the time a bit.

ourselves and our health. You notice that you are feeling a little overworked and overtired. And you've heard exercising can help but with this kind of schedule, who has time?

By committing to a walking program, you are killing two birds with one stone. Not only are you getting the exercise you need, you are also getting some time to clear your mind and to step away (literally) from the responsibilities of home, work, and/or school. It allows you to reflect upon the day's events—or not. Sometimes, just going out for a walk to empty the mind is all you need to feel replenished and revived. Whatever your reasons may be, taking a walk serves as a good excuse to escape the trials and tribulations of your everyday routine and allow yourself the freedom to let go for a few moments.

Clearly Clarifying

With all of this information coming in through television, magazines, the Internet, work, school, and people, you probably find yourself feeling pretty buzzed and over-stimulated all the time. In addition to this persistent stream of confusion, you feel this constant pressure to "keep up with the Joneses" (whoever they are) and to have the biggest and the best that America has to offer. No sooner have you conquered one goal than you're off trying to attack the next.

Setting aside time for a walk, even if it is just for 20 minutes, provides you a moment to pause and reflect about the information of the day. You need to put things in perspective and to process all this incoming information so that you can organize it in a coherent and comprehensive fashion in your mind. It gives you a chance to think things through without the distraction and noise of the office, the children, or your fellow students. Allowing yourself some time to clarify will make a world of difference in how you approach your work, your family, and your studies. You come back feeling refreshed, calmer, and more willing to concentrate and focus on the work in front of you.

I Want My Mother Nature!

Believe it or not, the earth was not created covered with cement and sprouting sky-scrapers. Beyond the "concrete jungle" are beautiful sequoias, vast green meadows, and rushing rivers. Mother Nature has an amazing amount of free beauty to offer and it is all just a walk away! Unfortunately, you're probably so busy you never get the chance to get out and enjoy it. Many of you get up before the sun rises and go to bed after it sets. You are indoors and breathing circulated air all day long.

Committing to taking a walk just one day per week, in the woods or a local park, is essential to maintaining some balance in your life. It helps to put your world in perspective and to realize that you have a whole lot out there besides deadlines and conference calls. The next time you are feeling stressed and overwhelmed, think back to that time when you stopped for a little shade from the sun under the vast branches of that 100-year-old redwood tree. It may not solve any of the issues at hand, but it might at least give you a little perspective.

Just Step Out Your Front Door and You Are on Your Way!

Just in case the mind, body, and soul benefits aren't convincing enough, let me add a couple more reasons why walking is an excellent means of exercise, one that you should be considering quite seriously by now. IT'S CHEAP! No gym membership, no parking-garage fees, and no fancy equipment gathering dust in the basement. All you really need is a good pair of shoes and you are on your way. Plus, it actually works. Walking is a very efficient form of exercise if you do it consistently and within the guidelines prescribed. The *American College of Sports Medicine (ACSM)* recommends exercising three to five days a week for 20 to 60 minutes at 60 to 85 percent of your heart-rate max.

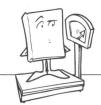

Weighty Words

ACSM stands for the **American College of Sports Medicine,** which is considered the institution with the "gold standard" for exercise prescription and instruction.

For All Walks of Life

Walking is also ageless, sexless, and timeless. Male or female, young or old, you can walk for however long you want. Many seniors are taking up walking as a means to improve overall health, including increasing their lung capacity, muscle endurance, and balance. Parents can let their tots run around silly to tire them out so that they will sleep through the night. And let's not forget about our social outings. Taking a walk with a friend, with your spouse and kids, or even with your boss are all opportunities to catch up on important issues and lost time while getting fit at the same time.

Walkers Watch Out!

The ACSM recommends that if you are over 40, have a medical condition, or have been sedentary for prolonged periods of time, you consult your physician before beginning an exercise program.

Easy as 1, 2, 3

Finally, walking is easy. Gone are the complicated instructions, expensive equipment, and assembly manuals. All you have to do is open your front door, and you're on your way! Adjusting walking to fit your needs is simple. If it's too hard, slow down. If it's too easy, pick up the pace. Need some variety? Walk on a trail, in the woods, or on the beach. It's raining? Try the treadmill. Need an event to compete in? How about a marathon or race-walking? Need a good cause (other than your own health)? You can find literally hundreds of walking events, nationwide and worldwide, raising money for anything from disease to saving the trees. So stop your excuses, lace up your walking shoes, and let's get going!

The Least You Need to Know

➤ Walking decreases depression, anxiety, and stress levels.

➤ Walking lowers your risk of heart disease, high blood pressure, and obesity.

➤ Taking a walk in nature once a week helps to clear your mind.

➤ Walking is one of the easiest and most efficient forms of exercise.

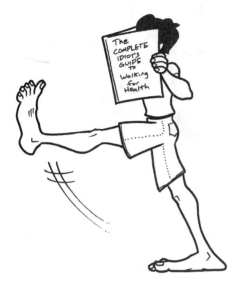

Chapter 2

One Step at a Time

In This Chapter

➤ Find out how to measure your fitness level

➤ What exactly does your heart rate tell you?

➤ Learn how to determine whether you are working hard enough

➤ Why speaking with your physician is important

So, you've decided that you would like to give this a try, huh? You don't exactly feel bad now, but you can see it coming and you'd like to do something about it. Great! But before beginning any fitness program, it is important to establish your starting point. Fitness testing is important because it gives you some objective feedback about your overall health. It also helps document how far you've progressed while determining certain areas that need special attention.

A complete fitness test involves cardiovascular (lung and heart), flexibility, and strength evaluations. It also includes an assessment of body composition (fat percentage) and girth measurements. In this chapter, I'll explain the various ways you can perform these tests on yourself. I will also help guide you through the process of understanding your heart rate, what it tells you, and how to use it to your advantage.

How Do You Measure Up?

Although we are a fat-fearing society, some fat is essential for our bodies to work properly. Fat serves as insulation to conserve body heat. It also helps protect your bones and internal organs. Lastly, it is a metabolic fuel for the production of energy. When you have not eaten enough, your body will turn to its fat stores for a little sustenance. Unfortunately, when *too* much fat is present in the body, you begin to put yourself at risk for disease. The following is a list of health conditions associated with obesity:

➤ Increased blood pressure

➤ Increased total cholesterol level

➤ Increased LDL (bad) cholesterol

➤ Increased risk of cardiac problems

➤ Increased risk of diabetes

➤ Hardening of the arteries

➤ Aggravation of osteoarthritis

➤ Increased predisposition to some cancers

➤ Decreased reaction time

➤ Reduced balance and coordination

➤ Increased susceptibility to infections

➤ Decreased circulation

➤ Delayed wound healing

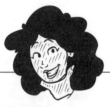

Interesting Excerpts

In a study of twins in which one sibling exercised and the other did not, those twins with higher levels of physical activity were associated with a lower total body fat, which suggests that exercise fights weight gain even in persons with a genetic predisposition to obesity.

—From *Reuters Health Annals of Internal Medicine 1999*, June 01, 2000

So, how do we determine whether you are over-fat? We measure you! There are several ways to measure your body fat. Some methods are more complicated than others and require special facilities and technicians, while others can be determined at home, by you the individual, with just a few simple calculations.

BMI

Your body mass index, or BMI, evaluates the healthfulness of your weight by measuring your height-to-weight ratio. The following are the simple calculations required for you to determine your BMI:

1. Determine your weight in kilograms (your weight ÷ 2.2 = W).

2. Determine your height in meters (height in inches ÷ 39.4 = H).

3. Multiply your answer to number 2 by itself (H × H) = H24. Divide your answer in number 1 by your answer in number 3 and you will have your body mass index: W × H2.

Once you've calculated the results, consult the following guidelines to determine where you stand in terms of standards established by the National Institutes of Health in 1999:

A BMI of 18.5 or lower is considered underweight.

A BMI between 18.5 and 24.9 is considered a healthy range.

A BMI of 25 to 29.9 is considered overweight.

A BMI of 30 or greater is considered obese.

Of course, there are other factors to consider besides height and weight that the BMI does not take into consideration, including muscle mass. Because muscle is denser than fat, it weighs more. Hence, a six-foot man with a lot of muscle mass will have much less fat than a six-foot man with little muscle mass who weighs exactly the same amount. They will also look very different. The more muscular man will be leaner and more compact than his fatter counterpart.

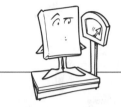

Weighty Words

Metabolic rate refers to the energy expended to maintain all physical and chemical changes occurring in the body.

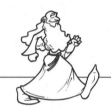

Wise Walkers

Body Mass Index is good for population-based studies and general guidelines, but not accurate enough from one individual to the next. If you do decide to measure your BMI, however, take into consideration the size of your ankles and wrists as well as your overall muscle density.

Waisting Your Hips Away: The Waist-to-Hip Ratio

The waist-to-hip ratio is a simple calculation that involves dividing the circumference of your waist by the circumference of your hips. Generally speaking, our hips are supposed to be wider than our waist. Unfortunately, this is not the case for everyone. In fact, recent studies have indicated that individuals with more middle-body fat (i.e., more fat in the torso) are at greater risk for heart disease than those whose fat is distributed below the waist. The reasons for this are not entirely clear, but it is believed that, with more fat closer to the chest, more pressure is exerted on the heart and it has to work harder to deliver blood to the rest of the body. Men whose waist-to-hip

Walkers Watch Out!

Watch your midsections. Studies show that fat around the waist is associated with an increased risk for chronic diseases such as diabetes and heart disease.

ratios are greater than one and women whose ratios are greater than .85 are at an increased risk for weight-related diseases.

Girth Measurements and Pants Size

Probably the most reasonable ways to determine whether you are overly fat are girth measurements and clothes size. Girth measurements are easy to calculate and reasonably accurate as long as you measure from the same place every time. You can measure just about any part of your body. Think of the areas where you put on weight the most. As mentioned earlier, some people carry more weight in their upper bodies while others let it all hang down. The following are some guidelines to help you with your measurements:

1. Start from the top down and always measure on the same side of the body (for example, if you measure the right side of the body, stay on the right side of the body).

2. Note the exact site you are measuring. Write it down so that subsequent measurements are accurate.

3. With the upper arm, measure the largest part of the arm between your shoulder and your elbow.

4. Measure your chest across your nipples.

5. For your waist, measure the narrowest part of your torso about an inch above your belly button.

6. For the hips, make sure you target the widest circumference across your bottom.

7. Like the arm, you should measure the thigh and the calf at the widest part.

Have a friend help you out, since holding the tape and accurately reading the numbers can be difficult. Needless to say, the fewer the clothes you have on, the better. Measuring against skin is going to be more accurate than against clothing. If for some reason you must take your measurements while clothed, remember exactly what you wear so you can wear the same thing the next time you take your measurements.

Of course, there is always the issue of clothing size. How many of us divide up our closets into fat clothes and skinny clothes? Even though it has been several years since you've fit into your "skinnies," you probably still keep them in the closet within eyes' view to remind you that you will *someday* fit into those size 6 Calvin Klein jeans, gosh darn it! Hang these on a hanger outside your closet door to serve as a reminder of your goals.

Scaling It Down

Let me take a minute to discuss scales here. As I mentioned above, scale weight can be very misrepresentative of someone's body-fat status. Too many people become a slave to their scales, allowing the daily number to dictate their moods from one moment to the next. Standard weight tables are based on very average statistics and do not take into consideration bone and muscle density. If you are going to weigh yourself, I offer the following suggestions:

➤ Do it at the same time of day every time.

➤ Weigh yourself using the same scale.

➤ Weigh yourself with as few clothes on as possible.

➤ Don't weigh yourself every day.

Also, keep in mind that your weight naturally fluctuates within a month, week, or even a day, particularly if you're female. Instead of taking the number on the scale so seriously, go by how you feel. Do you have more energy since you've started exercising? Are your clothes looser? Do you feel stronger and more confident in your skin?

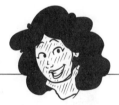

Interesting Excerpts

Although losing weight and getting in shape are excellent ways to improve your health, many people take it to the extreme and become obsessed with it. Being abnormally thin fits our society's current standards of beauty, which causes many people to feel overweight and unattractive when in fact they aren't either. This often leads to problems with self-esteem and self-image that can last a lifetime. Becoming aware of negative body image is important. There is an abundance of information available on improving your self-esteem at weightloss.about.com/health/weightloss/cs/bodyimage/.

My, How Strong and Flexible You Are!

Measuring your *muscle endurance* is an important factor in determining several things. First, it gives you some objective data from which to establish your goals. Second, it sets a starting point, to know how far you've come when you test again. Finally, it points out your weaker areas so you will know where to focus your attention. To keep things simple, I have listed four tests that focus on the main muscles of your upper

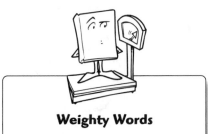

Weighty Words

Muscle endurance refers to the length of time that muscles can exert force continuously without fatigue.

and lower body. These are standard muscle endurance tests that will establish where you stand in relation to your own progress from one month to the next. All you will need is a timer and an exercise mat.

Upper Limits

Usually, when the words "push-up" are mentioned, images of drill sergeants and army barracks come to mind. That's because people in the military training camps actually do push-ups. The push-up is a very good gauge of upper-body strength. Not only are you working your chest and shoulders, you are also testing triceps, biceps, and stomach, as well as lower- and upper-back strength. One exercise that works all of those muscles? Pretty efficient, if you ask me. So now it's your turn; here's how you do it:

Lie on your stomach with your palms down, hands just in front of your shoulders. Keep your hips, shoulders, and neck in line as you raise your straight body off of the floor until the elbows are almost completely extended. Do not lock the elbows! Lower your weight slowly until your chest is about one to two inches from the floor. Repeat as many times as you can before the buzzer goes off.

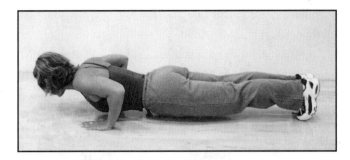

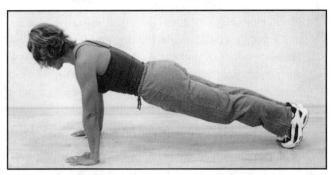

For those of you who feel a full push-up is not within the realm of possibility at the moment, keep your knees on the floor and raise your calves and feet. Remember to keep your hips, shoulders, head, and neck in line.

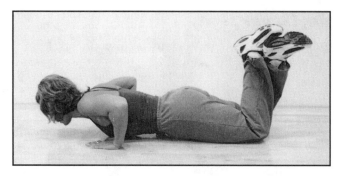

Lie on the floor face down. Place your hands under your shoulders and bend your legs at the knee, lifting your feet off the floor. With your hips, shoulders, and head in a straight line, bring your chest down so that it almost touches the floor then push back up.

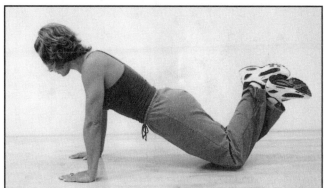

Results for Push-Up Test

Fitness Level Age	Poor	Fair	Average	Good	Excellent
Male					
<29	<20	20 to 34	35 to 44	45 to 54	>55
30 to 39	<14	15 to 24	25 to 34	35 to 44	>45
40 to 49	<11	12 to 19	20 to 29	30 to 39	>40
50 to 59	<4	5 to 9	10 to 19	20 to 29	>30
Female					
<29	0 to 5	6 to 16	17 to 33	34 to 49	>50
30 to 39	0 to 3	4 to 11	12 to 24	25 to 39	>40
40 to 49	0 to 2	3 to 7	8 to 19	20 to 34	>35
50 to 59	0 to 1	2 to 5	6 to 14	15 to 29	>30
>60	0	1 to 2	3 to 4	5 to 19	>20

The Lowdown on Your Lower Body

The next procedure involves testing the endurance of the muscles in your legs. Even though this is a static (immobile) test of leg strength and walking is a mobile exercise, it will still be helpful by giving you some indication of how strong your legs are when you start out.

Stand with your back against a wall, about two feet away from the base. Feet and knees should be about hips' width apart, toes pointing forward. Slide down against the wall until your upper legs are parallel to the floor. Make sure that you can see your toes and that your weight is on your heels. Hold this position for as long as you can or until you've reached a minute. Keep your knees at a 90-degree angle and make sure you can see your toes.

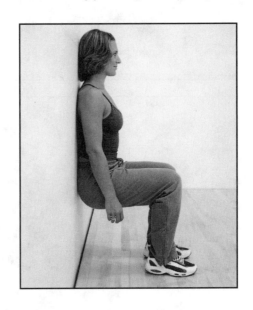

The following numbers will give you an idea of where you stand (no pun intended) with respect to leg strength:

Below average	<30 seconds
Average	30 to 60 seconds
Above average	>60 seconds

Wise Walkers

Remember to mark your results in a notebook so you will have it to refer to the next time that you evaluate your strength. Don't forget to include the date and the number of full push-ups you completed.

Stomach and Lower-Back Strength

Strong stomach and lower-back muscles are key to maintaining proper posture. They also help to reduce your risk of injury. Strong stomach muscles erect the spine, while weak ones curve it. There are many ways to test the muscles in your stomach and your lower back. Following, I have listed a couple of tests that are static, no movement, which are generally safer and easier to perform.

The first exercise is called the bridge and it focuses primarily on your stomach muscles with some emphasis on your lower back.

Walkers Watch Out!

If you have a history of knee pain or have had any surgery in the recent past, you should skip this test. Also, do not hold your breath! This raises your blood pressure and might cause you to faint.

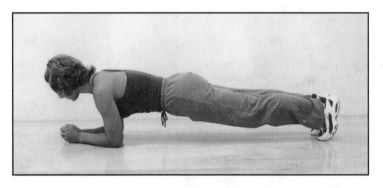

Lie on the floor face down. Place your elbows directly under your shoulders and clasp your hands together. Place your feet about hips' width apart.

Flex your feet with the tips of your toes on the ground. Lift your hips up so that all your weight is evenly distributed between your elbows and your toes.

Keep your stomach tight so that your back does not arch. Hold this position for as long as you can and record your result. Keep your head, shoulders, and hips in line and your back straight.

Below average: <10 seconds

Average: 10 to 30 seconds

Above average: 30 seconds or more

21

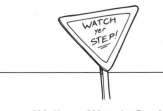

If you find that you cannot keep your back from arching, stop. Your stomach is not strong enough. This is a pretty fair warning that you will need to put some extra time into working your abdominal muscles. If you can hold the position from between 10 to 30 seconds, then you are "average" and in pretty good shape, but you still need to exercise regularly. Even if you're still holding the bridge and a minute has passed, you have above-average abdominal strength but you shouldn't stop your stomach exercises entirely, though you don't have to spend an inordinate amount of time on them, either.

The next test is essentially the same, but in reverse. This will test your lower-back endurance. Here is how you do it:

Lie on the floor on your back. Place your elbows directly beneath your shoulders. Place your feet about hips' width apart, with the back of your heels on the floor. With your back straight, lift your hips and hold for as long as you can. Again, record this number for future reference.

Keep your head, shoulders, and hips in line and your back straight.

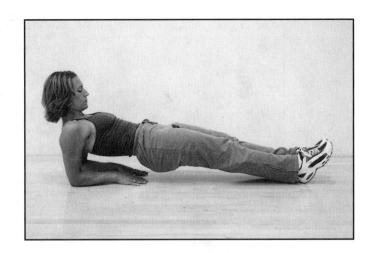

Below average:	<10 seconds
Average:	10 to 30 seconds
Above average:	30 seconds or more

Flexibility

How many of us have felt stiff getting out of bed in the morning? How about when we stand up from our desk or get out of the car after a long drive? This is a result of muscle tightness, which is caused by lack of movement of the joints. Flexibility is defined as the maximum ability to move a joint through its range of motion. Joint mobility is dependent on several things, including age, joint structure, and muscle tightness.

Because so many of us spend so much time sitting (and eating, watching TV, writing, reading, and working) our muscles may shrink and become tight. When we finally do move, they feel restricted and uncomfortable, which can cause a host of problems, including muscle tears and connective-tissue damage. Chronic pain in the lower back, neck muscles, and knees are just a few conditions associated with poor flexibility. Above and beyond the reasons already mentioned, here is a list of some other reasons why flexibility is so important:

➤ It increases circulation in the muscles and joints.

➤ It reduces muscle tension and fatigue.

➤ It increases your ROM, or range of motion.

➤ It enhances physical activity in general (sports and other).

➤ It improves muscle balance and posture.

To assess the flexibility of your ankles, sit in a chair with your feet out in front of you. Point and flex each foot as far as you can. Does one ankle feel easier to move than the other does? Next, place your feet flat on the ground and try to pick up just the arch of your foot, and then the outside of your foot. Again, note the differences between your ankles. Which one shows greater range of motion? Pay attention to these differences when you begin your walking program, since it is likely that the less-flexible foot might cause some problems down the road.

Having tight calf muscles can lead to shin splints and other problems. Keeping these muscles warmed up and flexible is an important factor in avoiding injury. Perform the exercise in the following figure to assess your calf flexibility.

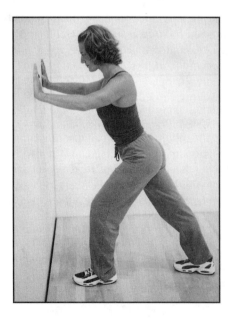

Stand an arm's length from a wall. Lean into the wall, bracing yourself with your arms. Place one leg forward with knee bent. No weight should be placed on this leg. Keep your other leg back with knee straight and heel down. Keeping your back straight, move your hips toward the wall until you feel a stretch. Hold for 30 seconds. Relax. Repeat with the other leg.

Note whether you can keep the heel of your straight leg on the ground. If not, your calves are probably pretty tight. Make sure you spend some extra time on them before you go out for your walk.

The hamstring is involved in almost every movement performed by the body. It is conveniently located at the back of your thigh and is responsible for bending the knee as well as kicking the leg back, two movements that are critical in walking. Having tight hamstrings is uncomfortable and can lead to a lot of lower-back pain and other injuries. To assess the flexibility of the hamstring, you can do what is known as the "sit and reach" test:

Sit on the floor with your legs straight out in front of you and your toes flexed. Start to bend forward at the hips, and try to touch your toes. Keep your back straight, and imagine trying to bring your stomach to your thighs.

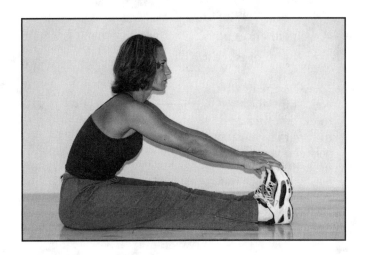

If you cannot straighten the back of your thighs onto the ground, your hamstrings' flexibility is below average, and you need to stretch them often. If your legs are straight and you can manage a slight bend at the hips, you've got average flexibility, but you will still need to spend a good amount of time stretching your hamstrings. If you can touch your toes and/or touch your head to your shins, you are above average and only need to maintain your hamstring flexibility.

Hip flexors are the muscles in front of your hips that bring the leg forward and pull the knee up. These are very important muscles for walking and are often very tight because of the amount of time we spend sitting (bringing the hip and thigh into a 90-degree angle shortens the hip flexor). Because the hip flexors connect to the spine, their tightness is often the culprit of lower-back problems. Walking can contribute to this tightness because of the repetitive motion of pulling the leg forward. Here is how you assess the hip flexors:

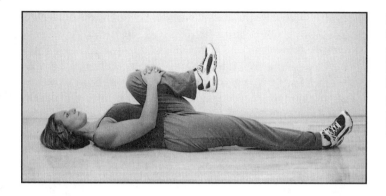

Lie on your back, both legs straight and on the floor. Bend one knee and bring it to your chest. Keep the other leg on the floor. To prevent your back from arching, press your lower back into the floor.

If you notice that your straight leg is lifting off the floor, foot included, the flexibility of your hip flexors is below average and you must stretch them daily if possible. If you can keep the foot of the straight leg on the floor, but the knee is slightly bent and there is a space between the floor and the back of the leg, your hamstrings are *less* tight, but you should still stretch them at least every other day. If you can press the back of the entire leg on the floor, then you have flexible hip flexors.

Your shoulders and back are also important muscles involved in walking. Even though the legs and the lower body are the primary movers in an exercise such as walking, the arms and the upper back play a large role in the efficacy and balance of the movement. Having a flexible upper body helps you to move with more ease. It also builds the momentum in your stride and helps to keep you balanced. The scratch-and-touch test is a good assessment of your shoulder flexibility:

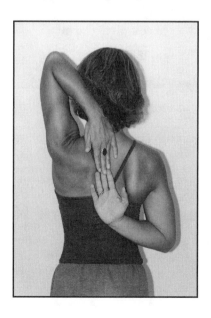

Stand with your feet hips' width apart. Bring one arm behind your back (palm facing out) and the other arm behind your head (palm facing your back). In the mirror (or with your fingers) see or feel how close your fingers come along the middle of the spine. Switch your arms and repeat.

If the fingers touch when you place your hands on your back, you have above-average shoulder flexibility. If you can bring your hands behind you but cannot connect your fingers, your shoulder flexibility is average and you will need to spend some time working to stretch them. If you can't even bring your hands behind your back, you have poor flexibility in your shoulders and you should definitely make it a priority to stretch at least every other day.

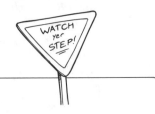

Walkers Watch Out!

Poor shoulder flexibility could cause tightness in your chest, leading to excess tension, and pull in the upper back an area where many people "carry their stress."

Knowing Your Cardiovascular Starting Point

The cardiovascular system is made up of the lungs, heart, and circulatory system. Its efficiency is measured by how easily these three components deliver oxygen and nutrients to the working muscles. The greater your cardiovascular endurance, the quicker and easier it is to deliver O_2 and energy to your muscles. The one-mile walk is a great way to test your cardiovascular endurance, since it is a timed distance test. and the best thing to do is to go to a local track to conduct this test. Begin by warming up for 5 to 10 minutes and proceed with two to five minutes of stretching. Once you feel ready, mark the time, get ready, set, and go! Walk the mile distance as fast as you can without stopping. When you've completed the mile, stop your watch and cool down for 5 to 10 minutes. You can write down two things: your heart rate and your time. Keep these numbers in a safe place so you can refer to them at your next test. The following table below indicates your fitness level by how long it took you to complete the mile:

Above average	Less than 13 minutes
Average	Between 13 and 15 minutes
Below average	15 minutes or longer/could not complete

There are always standards to which you can compare your results. knowing where *you* started individually (regardless of how fit or unfit you are in relation to the rest of the world) is important so you can refer back to it in time to see how far you've come.

The Importance of Understanding Your Heart Rate

Other than telling us that we are alive and kicking, the heart rate is also a monitor of how efficiently we are, or are not, training. A high resting heart rate, for example, indicates to us that we've been over-training and might need to take a day or two off. If, on the other hand, our resting heart rate drops a few beats in the morning, it is telling us that our heart is stronger and that we have improved our cardiovascular fitness.

Like any other muscle in our body, the heart becomes stronger with exercise. With the increase of physical activity, the heart must pump more blood and oxygen to the working muscle. Initially, this means that it has to pump faster to accommodate the increase energy. Over time, however, as the heart becomes stronger, it will grow in size, increase its *stroke volume,* and become more efficient at delivering blood to the muscles with fewer beats. Therefore, "cardiovascular fitness" is defined as the efficiency of the heart muscle and the lungs to not only deliver oxygen to the working muscles but also the efficiency of the muscles to absorb it.

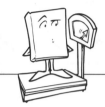

Weighty Words

Stroke volume refers to the amount of blood being pumped out of the heart per beat.

Heart Rate 1, 2, 3, 4

Here are four different ways to consider heart rate: The first is your resting heart rate, usually the lowest heart rate of the day, which you take before you get out of bed in the morning. On the opposite end of this scale is your maximum heart rate, or your highest pulse. Your maximum heart rate depends on how old you are, not on your fitness level, and is determined by subtracting your age from 220. Between these two is your target heart rate. The THR is the range of heart rates you should be working out in, and is based on a percentage of your maximum heart rate. Finally, there is your recovery heart rate. This is the timed pulse you take at the end of your workout. It helps to determine your overall fitness level as well as whether you need to adjust the intensity of your program.

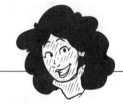

Interesting Excerpts

The more fit you become, the lower your recovery heart rate will be. That's because your heart doesn't have to work as hard as it did before you strengthened it through exercise.

Normal resting heart rates range between 60 and 80 beats per minute. The best way to measure your morning pulse is to do it from your bed, shortly after you wake up. As your cardiovascular system improves, your resting heart rate will decrease. A high resting heart rate, on the other hand, could be telling you that you are over-training and need a break. Try to take and keep track of your morning pulse regularly.

In order to increase your heart's strength, you need to push it harder than it is used to working for extended periods of time. Obviously, working it at its maximum capacity every time you exercise is inadvisable, not to mention probably impossible. Therefore, you must target your heart rate within certain percentages of its maximum capacity. This is what is known as your Target Heart Rate, or THR. Usually, in order to obtain the fitness benefits mentioned previously, it is recommended that you work at somewhere between 65 and 85 percent of your maximum heart rate. By keeping your heart rate within this range, you will not only work your heart hard enough to maximize the benefits of aerobic fitness, you will also keep it low enough so as not to overtax your cardiovascular system, which can lead to *over-training*.

Target Heart Rate Chart

Age	Max Heart Rate	Target Zone
20	200	130 to 150 to 170
25	195	126 to 146 to 165
30	190	123 to 142 to 161
35	185	120 to 138 to 157
40	180	117 to 135 to 153
45	175	113 to 131 to 148
50	170	110 to 127 to 144
55	165	107 to 124 to 140
60	160	104 to 120 to 136
65	155	100 to 116 to 131

In the preceding table, you will see that there are three numbers in the Target Zone. The smaller number is equivalent to a lower intensity workout while the larger number relates to the higher intensity range. The middle number is an average between the two (your target heart rate), which is equivalent to a medium intensity workout.

Recovery heart rate is also a strong indicator of your level of fitness. Most of us focus on the high numbers, when we are really mov'n and shak'n, but the lower numbers are equally important. Once you've finished your walk, during the cool-down, it is important to keep an eye (or your finger) on your pulse. The fitter you are, the faster your heart rate will drop. If your heart rate remains high during this recovery period, it is trying to tell you something, primarily that you need to take your intensity level down a notch or take a few days off.

Intensity and Heart Rate

Now that you understand what the different levels of your heart rate mean, you will need to know how to measure them. You can measure your heart rate in several ways. Some are simpler than others. Most of you are familiar with taking your pulse. This is the technique performed on you by the doctor or nurse every time you go for a physical. You can also determine your effort level by how hard/easy it is to talk while you are exercising. Finally, there is the heart-rate monitor, a funny little gadget that transmits the beat of your heart to a monitor that you wear on your wrist.

As I mentioned before, you can measure your effort level by palpation, or taking your pulse. You do this by placing your index and middle fingers just below your jaw line at the side of your neck. Get a regular pulse before you start. Set your watch and start counting the beats for 15 seconds. Multiply this number by four (15 seconds × 4 = 1 minute).

Another method of measuring the intensity of your workout is by evaluating how easy (or hard) it is to talk. Generally speaking (no pun intended, really), you want to push yourself to a level where talking is somewhat of an effort. You want to be able to carry on conversation, but with some difficulty, pausing to catch a couple of breaths to continue. If you cannot speak at all, you need to bring it down a notch; if you are having no trouble talking at all, you will need to pick up the pace a bit.

Finally, you might want to try a heart-rate monitor, which consists of a strap you hook around your chest that transmits electromagnetic waves from your heart to a monitor around your wrist. These are fun to have because you can actually see your heart rate rise and fall as you adjust your effort level.

There are all kinds of heart-rate monitors and they can get quite complex. Stick with the most basic model, the one that reads just your heart rate. They usually come with a little booklet that explains how to work the device, although it's pretty easy to figure out on your own. They are expensive, however, and are somewhat high-maintenance, as you usually will need to send the device back to the manufacturer for repairs.

Getting the Doctor's Okay

Finally, before beginning any exercise program, it is important to consult your doctor. Even though you may be young and healthy, it is advisable to at least drop him or her a line to let them know of your exercise plans. For those of you who are over 40, it is highly recommended that you speak with your doctor. If you are a smoker, have diabetes, a history of heart disease, high cholesterol, or have been sedentary for a long time, it is required that you get the okay from your physician before starting an exercise program. Even though exercise is good for most of you, it can be quite a dramatic change for your body when you first start out. Plus, you might need to be aware of certain modifications that only your doctor will be able to tell you about.

The Least You Need to Know

➤ Knowing where you started helps to determine where you should go.

➤ There are four levels of the heart rate with respect to fitness.

➤ Measuring your heart rate is easy and important.

➤ Checking with your doctor before beginning your program will help determine proper guidelines and safety.

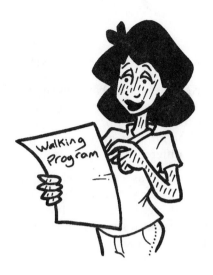

Beginning a Program

Congratulations! You've survived the basic instructions provided in Chapter 2, "One Step at a Time," and still want to find out more about walking. This is a good sign.

But the hard part is making a commitment to yourself, which is crucial to starting and staying with any exercise program. Knowing yourself and being honest about your strengths and weaknesses is key for your success. Finding the time to exercise, making it a habit, mapping out your goals, and rallying up a strong support system are the backbone for a sturdy program.

In this chapter, I'll help you create a practical routine. First, we'll scrutinize your appointment book and create time in your busy life to "fit it all in." Then I'll give you tips on how to anticipate the hard times as well as reward the good ones. Be proud of yourself for coming this far. Now I invite you to come join me to find out just how far you can go.

C Is for Commitment

Making a commitment to exercise is both the easiest and the hardest aspect of beginning a program. How many times have you sworn to get healthy but never followed through, or dropped off after just two or three weeks? Fitness clubs bank on the probability that their members will not exercise. They sell hundreds and even thousands of memberships that the gym, if everyone were to actually show up, would never be able to accommodate. Why is it that so many of us drop off after such a short amount of time, and how is this time going to be any different?

Most of us exercise to *look* better, with improving our health as a secondary goal. We all want to lose those extra 10 pounds, tone up the thighs for summer, or increase our chest size to make us look bigger. This is not a bad thing. With so much emphasis on image in this country, it is okay to want to look good. But it is also important to feel good. After all, how many sick people do you know who look vibrant and alive? Probably very few. Health equals vitality, and vitality is a very attractive trait to have. Without good health, we may as well forget about our good looks.

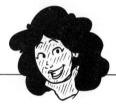

Interesting Excerpts

Research shows that diets are unsuccessful at producing long-term health and weight loss and control. Only five percent of people who go on diets are successful at losing the weight and keeping it off. The reason for this is that diets are quick fixes, temporary solutions that don't teach us how to change our poor eating habits, but in fact encourage them instead. Chances are that once you've lost the weight, it's only a matter of time before your return to your old patterns and gain the weight back again.

Take some time to educate yourself on the health benefits of exercise. The Internet is an amazing resource for all kinds of information and can provide a host of articles, links, and Web sites on health and the advantages of staying healthy. If you are without a computer, check out the health and wellness section at your local bookstore. You should be able to find any number of resources explaining the health benefits of exercise. Certain public radio stations and television shows have segments on health and exercise that are also very resourceful.

Once you've learned why exercise is so important, honoring your commitment and taking health seriously might seem a little easier. Make it a priority. If you tend to be a workaholic, remind yourself how stress can damage your health and how, if you do get sick, you might have to stop work entirely. If you are busy with kids and family duties, use your imagination to try to find ways to incorporate a little free time for yourself. Trade off with a neighbor or your spouse, hire a babysitter, or just take the kids with you. Keep exercise a priority and make an effort to overcome obstacles.

I know it is easy to lose focus, especially if the results are slow in coming. But if you are consistent, results will come. In the meantime, keep reminders of your goals accessible and within sight. Post a quote, a photo of you in healthier days, or some article with invigorating health statistics within eye view. Chase away negative thoughts as they are inevitably going to try to interrupt your progress. Tell yourself that they are just patterns of thinking that can be changed with a little effort and perseverance. Call a friend when you need some extra support; most people are happy to give you a little pep talk when asked.

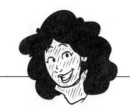

Interesting Excerpts

As Ralph Waldo Emerson said, "The first wealth is health."

Time Is of the Essence

If I could capture time in a bottle and sell it, I'd be a wealthy woman. Despite the technological advancements that allow us to save time, we have become increasingly busy. When people are asked why they don't exercise, they usually answer that they have "no time," or are "too busy," or "too tired." But you've just got to make the time to exercise. So, let's start with the calendar and the appointment book. First, try to eliminate the things that you absolutely can do without—nail appointments and *Ally McBeal* episodes included. Next, try to organize your time more wisely. Combine errands and schedule appointments in blocks. Next, make an appointment with yourself to exercise. Mark it in permanent black ink so it cannot be erased. Tell your assistant to keep your appointment standing no matter how much you "must" change it a week later. Look into the future to apprehend and work around obstacles. Plan ahead and be organized. By doing this, you will avoid excuses that inevitably arise at some time.

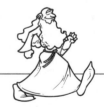

Wise Walkers

Make a standing date to exercise with a spouse, friend, or co-worker. Agree that you will help motivate each other and not back out of your commitment, no matter what.

Make Walking a Habit First

So much information is out there about walking and exercise that it can be overwhelming. How fast to walk, how long, how many days, percentage of heart-rate max, rate of perceived exertion—it can be exhausting just trying to process it all. Even though you can learn a lot of useful and important information, probably the most important is that walking must become a habit first!

Walking is a state of mind as much as it is an exercise. You have to start thinking of yourself as a walker in order for it to stick. For many people, especially those who have never exercised, this is a difficult task. If you have not thought of yourself as the athletic type, it is hard to suddenly imagine yourself as an exerciser. So take it slow. Start by taking it one day at a time. Commit to two 10-minute walks a week. Don't worry about your heart rate or your route right now, just make sure you step out your front door and move around for a few minutes. Build up the confidence slowly. After two to three weeks of walking twice a week, add another day to the routine.

Even if you've been exercising all along but are new to walking, take it slow. The body needs time to adjust to the different demands on it. This is what is referred to as the *specificity* of training meaning: Your body adapts uniquely to the specific types of strain being put on it. For example, if you've spent the last 10 years running and working your legs, chances are when you jump in the pool for a swim, even though you are in good shape, you will feel a little winded. This is because the bulk of your effort in the pool comes from your upper body.

Exercise is a way of life and not just a temporary fix to drop a few pounds or tone up your legs for summer. Even though these are good motivators to start a program, it is important to start thinking of walking as a lifestyle change, something you will do as long as you can. You must continue to challenge your body if you want to continue to reap the benefits of exercise. Reaching your goal and stopping will only lead to slipping behind and having to start all over again.

Just accept that walking is now part of your life—something you do because you have to, like eating breakfast or going to work. If you miss a day or even a month, you can get back to it. The all-or-nothing way of thinking can be very detrimental in establishing healthy habits. Remember that substantial changes are slow, so take your time accepting it as a lifestyle change rather than as a temporary solution.

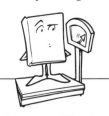

Weighty Words

The principle of **specificity** states that only those systems that are emphasized will adapt and change.

Wise Walkers

Make walking nonnegotiable. For example, if you debate with yourself about exercising every morning, you'll probably opt for staying in bed for another half an hour. But if getting up for exercise is no more negotiable than getting up for work, then you'll do it regardless of how you feel about it.

Establishing Long- and Short-Term Goals

Establishing goals is a very important part of a successful walking program. Goals help you stay focused and motivated. They remind you why you are doing what you are doing. Without a clear set of goals, you lose the sense of purpose that can make your exercise attempts seem useless. Usually, in the beginning we all start out very optimistic and hopeful. This time we are really going to get fit. Come Monday, we are ready to go. Walk! Walk! walk … walk … walk … walk … okay, this is getting a little tiresome *and* boring! Why the heck am I out here circling the block in the pouring rain when I could be inside on the sofa, watching *Friends?* Setting both short- and long-term goals prevents you from losing your direction.

Write down your fitness goals. Don't worry about their order; just scribble them down as they come to you. Next, take a closer look at the list. Be honest with yourself and cross off those that aren't realistic or obtainable. Then, try to be as specific as possible with each goal. If, for example, your top priority is to lose weight, specify what you mean exactly. Do you want to lose 5 pounds or 10 pounds? Do you want to be able to fit into that red summer dress by June? Once you've broken down your goals into more detail, set a date for the first one on your list. Again, be realistic. Losing 10 pounds in two weeks is possible, but definitely not healthy. Give yourself a reasonable amount of time so you don't run into disappointment and frustration because you didn't accomplish what you wanted to in the time frame you allotted.

If Only … Long-Term Goals

Long-term goals are those that you have always wanted to meet, but just haven't been able to manage. In order to be successful in meeting long-term goals, you must be very careful about which ones you choose. First and foremost, they must be realistic. If, for example, you have a bum knee, it might not be a good idea to set your sites on running a marathon. Long-term goals should also be relatively specific and simple. Some examples of realistic, clear long-term goals might be to walk a 10K within a year, or to walk a mile in less than 10 minutes within six months.

Breaking Down and Getting Down: Monthly and Weekly Goals

Long-term goals are too overwhelming to focus on all the time. They are too far away and may seem insurmountable at first. That's why you should break down your goals into smaller, more obtainable, short-term goals. Monthly and weekly goals are easier to aim for and to tackle, as long as you're

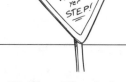

Walkers Watch Out!

Don't feel bad if you adjust your goals. Redefining your goals does not mean that you've failed—only that you've learned from your experience.

realistic in setting them. If your goal were to cut a 17-minute-mile walk into a 13-minute-mile walk, you'd do best to try increasing your speed by half a mile per minute every month for a year. If you exercise three to five times a week, pushing your speed on two of those days, you'll soon be meeting your long-term goal by meeting some short-term ones along the way.

One Day at a Time: Daily Goals

Daily goals are even more specific. Using the example above, a daily goal might be to alternate walking two blocks more slowly with walking three blocks quickly on each of your two "pace" days.

But don't be too strict. This can cause more damage than good. Setting expectations that are too high often leads to frustration and disappointment and can cause you to drop off entirely from your routine. Again, be realistic; look at your week and adjust your goals accordingly. You might have had to work overtime all week and not gotten enough sleep. Pushing your pace under these circumstances would be detrimental. Take a break and make up for the lost time the following week. Here is a summary of the long- and short-term breakdown:

➤ **Year's goal:** Walk one mile in 10 minutes (current time 17 minutes).

➤ **Monthly goal:** Subtract 30 seconds from time every month.

➤ **Weekly goal:** Walk four times a week/push pace two days.

➤ **Daily goal:** Subtract eight seconds from each of the weekly "pace" walks.

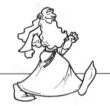

Wise Walkers

Start saving money for your treats now. Have a box or a piggy bank that you drop a little bit of money into each time you accomplish something you are proud of.

Reveling in Rewards

Remember: All work and no play makes Jack a dull boy. You deserve some praise and gratification for all your hard work. Write a list of guilty pleasures—activities or treats you normally consider too indulgent. Organize them so that the more costly and time-consuming ones are at the top. Write your goals in the next column, placing your toughest long-term goal next to the best reward.

Every time you accomplish a goal, reward yourself. Again, be realistic. If you're trying to lose weight, don't choose a hot fudge sundae as your reward. Some examples of your smaller rewards might be treating yourself to a facial, a massage, or a new pair of shoes. For your bigger accomplishments, you could plan a trip to Hawaii or some health spa or go on a shopping spree. Be careful and budget yourself wisely. The following are some tips on how to increase your chances of successfully achieving your goals:

➤ Be realistic: Your goals should be attainable.

➤ Measure your progress regularly.

➤ Set realistic dates. Don't be overambitious, because this can set you up for disappointment and failure.

➤ Write everything down so you can review it.

➤ Reward yourself for every goal achieved.

Building a Support System

Another very important aspect of success other than goals and rewards is support. Perhaps this is the most important aspect of your commitment. Take the time to tell those closest to you what your plans are. Ask them for their help. Make a small list of your areas of weakness and devise some plans to deal with them as they arise so you will be prepared. Gather a list of inspiring quotes, poems, articles, and photographs and paste them in obvious places around your home and work. Be proactive and committed.

Telling your family members and co-workers about your plan is a good idea. They will be more likely to ask you about your progress and put some healthy pressure on you to keep up your commitment. People commonly start out really motivated, but this enthusiasm is bound to dwindle over time. By telling other people, you have committed to someone other than yourself and backing out is less easy. Ask for specific help from those closest to you. For example, if you tend to go all out when dining with your wife and your goal is to lose weight, ask her to remind you gently of your commitment before you order the nachos with extra cheese. A co-worker might agree to send you a motivational e-mail or drop you a voicemail if you need her to. Be honest with yourself and ask for all the help you need.

Joining a walking group is another excellent source of support. Although the idea might be somewhat intimidating at first, it can be a very good move. For one, you will be meeting people who are in the same shoes as you (almost literally), who can help you get through the harder times. Second, chances are that you will come across someone who shares

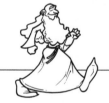

Wise Walkers

Here is an online resource for those of you who like to chat via the Internet: The Walking Chat. We chat each weeknight for an hour, starting at 6 P.M. PST, 7 P.M., 8 P.M., and 9 P.M. Check it out at walking.about.com/ recreation/walking/mpchat.htm.

a similar story to yours, and who can offer good advice on ways to improve your program and overcome challenges. It's also a good way to find new areas to walk. A group of people is a better resource than just one person. It's safer, too. Attacking a group of walking wonders is unwise, and the prowlers know it. Finally, it serves as an excellent and healthy social-networking system. It's a way to meet new people who share common interests and values. If you are new to the area or have recently gone through a divorce, this might be an excellent way to meet new friends.

The Least You Need to Know

➤ True commitment is key to starting and maintaining a new walking program.

➤ Finding the time in your busy life is half the battle.

➤ Creating new habits are the steppingstones for consistency.

➤ Setting realistic goals is essential for keeping focused and determined.

➤ A good support system is a sure way to keep the commitment to yourself and to others.

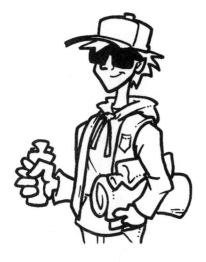

Gathering Your Gear

Now comes the fun part ... shopping!! Although you'll need a few things to start your walking program, you certainly won't need to buy out the store, and you'll want to guard against being convinced by eager clerks to do just that. In this chapter, I will explain some of the different types of materials that are available and which ones might be more appropriate for certain environmental conditions than others. I will also discuss some of the "things" you can (and should) take along with you to ensure a safe, injury-free, comfortable, and fun walk.

Comfort vs. Style: Making the Right Clothing Choices

I admit it: I am definitely caught up in the whole fashion fitness thing. I like to color-coordinate and wear the most "in" workout gear. But my fashion follies only go so far. The worst thing is being too preoccupied with some uncomfortable piece of clothing

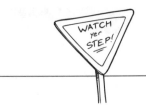

to enjoy your workout. So, I draw the line on fashion when discomfort enters the picture. It is more important to be comfortable than to be stylish. Whatever your fashion preferences, you should consider some important factors when shopping for walking gear. For example, is layering really necessary? What are all these new materials out there and how in the heck do you pronounce their names? Does tight clothing have some advantage over loose clothing, or vice versa? Are shorts better than pants? And what about supportive gear, for her *and* for him?

Lotsa Layers

Because your body will experience changes in temperatures at the beginning, middle, and end of your walk, you might want to consider wearing your clothing in layers. Exercise raises your body temperature. Your muscles, lungs, and heart are all working harder to accommodate the increase of activity being demanded on them. Your body will begin to sweat in an attempt to keep itself cool. If all you have on is a big wool sweater, chances are that you are going to spend the majority of your walk uncomfortable and frustrated. And how about at the end of your walk? The purpose of the cool-down is just that: to "cool down" and bring your body temperature back to normal. If you're only wearing a little cotton T-shirt, you'll start to feel wet and cold as you near the end of your walk, which is not only uncomfortable but also unhealthy.

Finally, you must consider the very likely fact that your environment will vary depending on the terrain, on the time of day, and on the weather. Mornings tend to be cooler than afternoons, for example. Mountains are usually windier than flatlands and the weather, depending on where you live, can vary from one hour to the next. Be proactive and check your local forecast. Layering your clothing will help you adjust to different internal and external conditions.

With all of this in mind, your first layer of clothing should be made of a fabric able to absorb sweat. Sweat helps to maintain a healthy body temperature. If you wear a piece of clothing that prohibits your skin from releasing moisture in a hot environment, then you are putting yourself at risk for overheating. Likewise, in cooler weather, if you are wearing a garment that doesn't absorb the sweat from your skin, you could become hypothermic.

You also want to choose as a first layer a material that insulates you while allowing your skin to breathe. Some amazing new fabrics are out there these days. Many of them are mixed-synthetic materials that have multipurpose functions. You want to choose a garment that "wicks" the moisture from your body. Wicking refers to the capability a material has to not only sponge the water from your skin, but also transfer the moisture through the clothing and into the atmosphere. Most of these specialty fabrics are sold at mainstream athletic stores, such as Big 5 and Copeland's. If you decide you want to check it out, keep your eye out for key words such as *Polypropylene*, CoolMax, and a polyester/cotton mix.

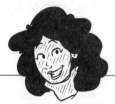

Interesting Excerpts

The body is made up of over 75 percent water. Water helps to regulate our body temperature through sweating. Sweating is the body's natural cooling system. Your body's health depends on its ability to release and absorb water through hydration and perspiration. If you do not drink enough water, or if you wear clothing that does not allow your body to release sufficient heat through sweating, you are at risk for heat illness and other heat injuries. Make sure you wear clothing that allows your skin to breathe and maintain its normal system of temperature control.

Your second layer should be made of a fabric capable of insulating you, keeping you warm as you prepare your muscles for increased movement. I suggest fleece because it insulates heat and retains body warmth—it's also comfy. There are two types of fleece: synthetic (polar) fleece and Eco fleece. Synthetic fleece comes in different weights that coincide with their intended use. Heavier fleece (300) is used for colder environments while lighter fleece (100) can be used for moderate temperatures such as spring mornings or fall afternoons. Eco fleece is a newer material and is made out of recycled plastic bottles. Environmentally conscious manufacturers decided to use existing material rather than adding to the waste of the world and came up with the Eco fleece idea. Your last layer should be some sort of shield that protects you from the elements and should be both waterproof and windproof. Walking in the rain can be fun when wearing the proper gear.

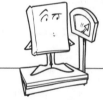

Weighty Words

Polypropylene is a material exhibiting excellent seam strength and resistance to cold-flow with form-fitting and flexible properties, that can be used in strong sunlight because of its excellent UV/weathering/ozone resistance.

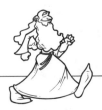

Wise Walkers

Remember that walking above certain elevations means that you will have less oxygen (air) to breathe, which will make you more winded. If you are taking a trip to a mountainous hideaway, check out the elevation just so you are prepared.

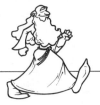

Wise Walkers

Size is important here. Loose or tight, make sure you pick the correct size. Wearing the wrong size will distract you from your walk.

Choose materials that are water resistant but that also enable your body to release heat and to breathe. Gore-Tex is a good name to remember when shopping for jackets and windbreakers. Nylon is another material to consider, especially for those windier walks.

Hang'n Loose

With respect to the issue of tight vs. loose clothing, I think it all depends on your own preference. For example, I prefer to wear clothing that is fairly form-fitting. I don't like my legs to jiggle because it distracts me from enjoying my workout. Also, looser clothing tends to gather in weird places so I end up spending the entire time readjusting it rather than enjoying my workout. However, you may feel much more at home in a baggy pair of pants. If you are layering up, you might want to make the first layer form-fitting and the other two loose to avoid too much bunching. Whatever your preference, comfort, again, is the emphasis.

Bear in mind that different materials fit differently. Some clothes are less giving than others and may require that you buy them baggy. Other materials are stretchy and adjustable and allow more room for flexibility. You don't necessarily have to stick just with "walking gear" per se. Walking in a comfortable pair of jeans or a loose skirt wouldn't be the end of the world (in fact, millions do it everyday). But be practical: Taking a stroll in one of those little thong leotards or a tight mini-skirt will not only be very uncomfortable, but may have you running (from a bunch of lookers) sooner than you are ready.

The Long and Short of Things

Choosing to wear shorts instead of long pants is also an individual preference. Some people insist on wearing shorts no matter what the weather. Having bare legs feels very natural and comfortable—plus, you get to work on your tan. If you are a shorts-strutter, make sure that the shorts do not gather as you walk, as this can cause the skin on the inside of your thighs to rub together and can be very uncomfortable, especially on long hikes. Leg width is also important when buying shorts. If the shorts are too tight, they can restrict both your movement and the blood flow to your legs and feet. Don't be afraid to wear the clothing around in the store a bit before purchasing anything. Do some deep knee bends and wide strides to test the size.

Long pants protect your legs from the elements, such as bugs, the sun, and branches with prickly thorns. They also help to warm you up a little faster than wearing shorts will. Make sure the pants you choose aren't too big, however. Pant legs that are too long can be a drag (literally) and can increase your risk of tripping or falling. Similarly, pants that are too small can hinder your stride and, like a tight pair of shorts, cut off the circulation in your legs. Again, make sure you test the garment first by walking around the store before you purchase anything.

Walkers Watch Out!

Before you buy anything, read the "care" instructions first. Some material can be very high-maintenance with complicated cleaning instructions or can require dry cleaning.

Sports Bras and Other Supportive Gear

Support for our more sensitive parts is key to comfortable walking. Hanging loose and fancy-free is a concept that disappeared with the 1970s. Even though walking is a relatively low-impact sport, it can shake the body up a bit—especially if you are walking fast. Take the time to invest in some good support gear. Make sure that the material absorbs sweat and, if possible, has wicking capabilities. Cut off annoying labels, as they are often the culprits of chaffing and uncomfortable rashes.

For women in particular, finding the right sports bra is crucial. Inadequate support is not only uncomfortable but can cause stretching of the skin around the breast. You want a bra that provides adequate support while allowing you to breathe. If the strap around your rib cage is too tight, you will find too much pressure exerted on your diaphragm. This may not only constrict your breathing, but also cause painful rashes and sores. Likewise, the straps over your shoulders should be wide enough, between a half-inch to an inch wide, so they don't dig into your skin. Many sports bras cross in the back, helping to distribute the weight evenly. Finally, if you're not intending to wear anything over the bra, make sure you buy something that doesn't look like lingerie.

And how about you guys? Inadequate support can be very uncomfortable and painful, not to mention embarrassing! Many shorts provide a lining that is usually sufficient support. Unfortunately, long pants are often without lining. Regular briefs, jock straps, or a pair of running shorts are some

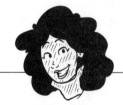

Interesting Excerpts

The first jogbra was invented in 1977 by Hinda Miller, who sewed two jock straps together and tied them around her chest area to provide more support to her breasts. Women loved the concept and the market for sports bras grew rapidly from that moment on.

suggestions to wear under your pants to add extra support. Or you can choose tights. Running tights serve two functions: Not only are they great for support, but they keep you warm, too. If you are too self-conscious to wear these in public, however, try wearing a pair of shorts or a loose pair of running pants over them.

Material Madness: Are Some Better Than Others?

Our technological advancements have brought a whole new type of synthetic clothing to our consumer fingertips. We have materials that absorb sweat, transfer heat, insulate core temperatures, wick moisture away, breathe, and practically do your laundry for you. But getting caught up in the mumbo jumbo of jumpsuit jargon is tiring and unnecessary. I will briefly summarize the components of a few of these "new" (and old) fabrics to help guide you in your search for walking clothes. Just remember that a lot of the lingo you read on labels is just a tool merchandisers use to make their garments sound "specialized" in order to try to convince you to buy their products. Keep it simple (and relatively cheap) and you should be fine.

Cotton Basics

What can be simpler and more comfortable than a pair of old sweats and a T-shirt? There is nothing wrong with sticking to the basics. Cotton feels comfortable on the skin and is both flexible and durable. A personal trainer by profession, I live in cotton sweats and find them to be the most comfortable clothing around.

But for exercise, cotton can be a drag, literally. As your body increases its energy output and your temperature rises, you begin to sweat. Cotton absorbs and holds on to this excess water. Unfortunately, it takes a long time for it to dry so you are likely to spend the majority of your workout in damp clothing. Needless to say, this can be very uncomfortable, heavy, and sometimes very cold (not to mention stinky). Therefore, although it is inexpensive and cozy, cotton may not be the most appropriate material for walking.

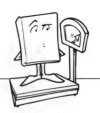

Weighty Words

The **gluteus maximus muscles,** a.k.a. buttocks, are very powerful. They come as a pair and make up two of the largest muscles in your body. Given this fact, you might need a little extra support to prevent too much wiggle (and jiggle).

Lycra: The Stretchy Stuff

Lycra is a stretchy fiber that moves easily with the body, providing maximum comfort, mobility, and shaping. It is also highly durable and flexible, and allows garments to retain their original shape. I tend to wear Lycra because it seems to hold everything in place—in particular, the *gluteus maximus,* or the buttocks. Nothing gathers and drags, so I feel more freedom of movement. Lycra is best used for your lower-body garments such as tights or shorts and is most comfortable as your first layer. Choose Lycra that is not made out of cotton, since cotton takes such a long time to dry. Look for Supplex Lycra, which is made out of nylon and is quick-drying.

Know'n Nylon

Nylon helps to shield the body from the wind. Many windbreakers are made of nylon. Clothing made from nylon tends to be loose and light so it is easy to move in. It also keeps some heat in. Many athletes wear nylon pants over their shorts or tights to speed up their warm-up. It dries quickly when wet, which makes it good to wear in the rain or snow. Unfortunately, nylon doesn't keep you warm, and it tends to suffocate the skin, keeping sweat in, rather than allowing the skin to breathe. Some nylon sweatsuits have cotton liners, which help a bit with sweat absorption and warmth retention. Wear it on top as a third layer and not as a layer that you put close to your skin.

CoolMax and Polypropylene

CoolMax and polypropylene are high-tech materials known as moisture-transport fabrics that serve to "wick" sweat away from the body. As you increase your activity level, your internal temperature rises and your body will automatically start to sweat in an attempt to cool itself down. CoolMax is 100 percent polyester and wicks moisture away from the skin and promotes evaporation. It has 20 percent more surface area than ordinary fibers to enhance moisture transfer. Polypropylene is a thermoplastic fiber that also serves to absorb and wick moisture away from the body. Many of these specialty garments are costly, however, and upkeep can be high maintenance. For a complete list of specialty fabrics, try the technical fabric glossary online at Totally Outdoors of Adventure Sports.

Shopping Resources

You can find an amazing amount of information available online. Don't get too hung up on clothing (no pun intended). I suggest shopping (live) in some local stores. Try on different types of clothing and materials. Don't be embarrassed to move freely, pick your knees up, squat down, kick back, and twist around while you are in the store trying to decide. Make sure the size is right and ask the store clerk for help if needed.

If you decide you do want to shop online, the Internet can be a very useful tool. About.com is, in particular, a very resourceful Web site for many things related to walking. If you go to their walking site, you will find, in the left-hand corner, an entire list of subjects ranging from gear and clothing to tours and treks. If you have access to the Internet and would like to check out About.com, this is what you need to do:

1. Type in www.about.com.

2. At the top, type in "walking" where it says "Find it now."

3. The third option down (Walking Site) is one of the resources I found most helpful.

4. The left-hand corner of this page has a list of subjects related to walking.

Following is a short list of some additional sites I explored for walking gear: The Walking Company, InSport, Title 9 Sports, and Wickers. If you do not have access to the Internet, you can find stacks of walking, running, and fitness magazines that usually provide a whole host of resources for clothing in the back of each issue. Check out your local shopping mall for stores specializing in athletic gear. Flip through the local newspaper and the Yellow Pages for advertisements. In addition, refer to Appendix A, "Resources for Walking Fit," for a list of companies and their addresses to help get you started.

Accentuating Accessories

How many of you feel "naked" without your Walkman? Everywhere you look these days you see exercisers, walkers included, with their headphones on. You might notice, too, that (if you're outside, in particular) they've got their sunglasses and hats on as well. Accessories are not necessities, but they are fun to experiment and play with. Certain accessories, however, are recommended to keep your walk safe, comfortable, and entertaining. In the following section, I will list some of the more important (and common) gadgets you should consider taking with you before you step out the door.

Walkers Watch Out!

Even though walking with a Walkman is a great way to make your walk sail by, be very careful about your surroundings. Make sure you can hear what is going on around you. Keep your eyes open and stay alert. Finally, never walk at night with your Walkman. People prey on those who are seemingly unaware and off in their own world.

Musical Moments

For some of you, music is the only way you are going to get through your workout. Without it you feel bored, anxious, and unmotivated. Music can be a great addition to your walking program. Not only can it make the time seem to go by faster, but it also adds a certain spring to your step. In my search, I found Sportsmusic.com to be a great resource for exercise music on tape. They provide a set of guidelines that help match the level of walker with the pace of music. They also offer a wide variety of music to choose from, depending on your style preference.

Of course, you can always choose your own music or make your own CDs and tapes if you don't want to spend the money. Remember, however, that CDs tend to skip, which can compromise your walking routine as you try to walk lighter to decrease the skipping; so make sure you have a fairly skip-less player if you are going to go the CD route.

Sensible Sun Block

"I'm just going to be out for an hour. It's not even sunny outside." Famous last words, as you wake up the next morning unable to even brush your teeth because your cheeks are so sunburned they feel like they are going to crack. The intensity of our sun is incredibly strong these days. All this talk about the ozone layer and global warming is true! And we must take every precaution to protect our skin from the sun's damage. So lather up before you go out. Wear SPF that is at least 15 or stronger. Make sure you get those forgotten places like on top of and behind the ears, and reapply when you've sweated excessively. Here are some guidelines to follow when walking in the sun:

➤ Choose a sunscreen that is at least 15 SPF.

➤ Apply the sunscreen before you go outside so your skin has time to absorb it.

➤ Don't forget the hard-to-remember places like your ears, back of the neck, and knees (and your bald spot if you have one).

➤ Reapply your sunscreen if you have been sweating or are out for a longer duration.

➤ Wear a hat and long sleeves if you are extra sensitive to the sun, to provide added protection.

Sight for Sore Eyes

Protecting your eyes is also very important. The sun's damage is not merely skin-deep. Over time, constant exposure to the sun can cause damage to your sight. In addition, you can see better when you're not squinting, so the risk of tripping and falling is less likely with proper eyewear. Make sure you find glasses with adequate UVA and UVB protection. Generally speaking, a good pair of sunglasses will cost at least $50. If you pay less, you might be buying a product with insufficient sun protection, so remember that you get what you pay for.

"You Can Leave Your Hat On"

Hats keep your head cool (and warm) when needed. They also help to shade your face from the sun and your eyes from the brightness. Make sure the hat fits comfortably on your head. If it is too small, it may constrict blood flow and cause discomfort. Loose hats fly away easily, and although running around chasing your hat might be considered exercise, it isn't exactly what I had in mind. Visors and baseball hats are good since the size can easily be adjusted. Try to find a hat that incorporates a sweat-band around the rim to prevent sweat from dripping into your eyes. Straw hats are cool-looking and functional, but can be scratchy on the forehead after some time. If you do wear a straw hat, wear a bandanna underneath to prevent an uncomfortable rash from forming on your forehead.

Band-Aids for Blisters

Although I will be covering the topic of minor and major injuries in another chapter, I would like to explain briefly why a box of Band-Aids is an important addition to your accessory list. Even though your feet feel good and your shoes fit well, you are not immune to blisters. Repetitive motion for long periods of time, even in the best of shoes, can cause wear and tear on your toesies. How many times have you begun a walk only to have to turn around early and limp home because of a blister? Blisters are fluid-filled sacs caused by heat and friction. Because they are on your feet, and because it is a requirement that we wear shoes almost everywhere we go, blisters take a long time to heal due to the constant irritation of having something rub against them all of the time.

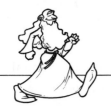

Wise Walkers

You can find standard Band-Aids at most large grocery stores or pharmacies. Shopping hint: Don't look for these in the bandage aisle, but in the foot-care section.

Band-Aid now has "Blister Block" cushions that help protect your feet from blisters. Dr. Scholl's also carries "Cushlin blister pads" to help prevent irritation. These are self-adhesive and they stick mightily to the skin—and can stay there for days if needed. You might want to consider investing in some of these blister busters to keep your feet pain-free and happy.

Walking with a Big Stick

The traditional image of the weathered walker usually involves a long beard, some grubby trousers, and a big walking stick. Rugged macho men surviving in the wild wilderness with the bare essentials may be the romantic image of the past, but it is no longer a requirement to carry a walking stick.

Some people grow very fond of their walking sticks and spend a great deal of time caring for them. But do they have a functional purpose? Are they helpful? Actually, yes. Other than helping you hoist yourself up hills and rocks, they assist you in maintaining balance and stability. Some have even been used to ward off large, hairy mammals and small, slimy reptiles as well. Walking sticks are not what I'd categorize as necessities, but they are useful and can be an amazing display of craftsmanship. If you are interested in finding out more about walking sticks, try Whistle Creek, PO Box 580, Monument, CO 80132; phone 719-488-1999. They have some helpful hints as well as amusing customer input regarding choosing a walking stick.

The Watered Walker

The human body is made up of more than 70 percent water. Water cools us down and maintains proper body temperature. It is also imperative for the functioning of healthy cells and the maintenance of electrolyte balance. Finally, water boosts our energy and keeps the body running smoothly. Try to drink at least eight cups of water daily. If you are active, or you live in a hot environment, you must drink even more water to stay caught up. Try to drink water before, during, and after your walk. You must replace two cups of water for every pound lost from sweating.

Drink small bits at a time to avoid cramps when you are walking. Remember that caffeine is a diuretic and increases fluid loss. Try to drink two glasses of water for every caffeinated beverage you drink. Always bring a bottle of water with you on your walks. It isn't necessary to buy a new bottle each time, either. Fill up your old bottle with filtered water from the tap. In fact, save your old water bottles, fill up a few at a time, and store them in the refrigerator to keep them cool.

Walkers Watch Out!

Drink water before you feel thirsty. Feeling thirsty is the body's signal to you that it is already dehydrated and needs water. Dehydration can cause fatigue and even kidney failure, so try to be diligent about your re-hydration. Generally speaking, you should drink at least eight large glasses of water a day and even more if you are active or if you consume a lot of caffeinated or alcoholic beverages. Certain foods like fruits and vegetables are high in water content so increasing your dose of them is a good idea.

The Least You Need to Know

➤ Feeling comfortable while you walk is very important.

➤ The correct choice of material depends on the environment in which you walk.

➤ Be specific when shopping for your walking gear.

➤ Accessories are fun and important for a healthy, successful walk.

Part 2

Progressing Safely

Be proud of yourself! You've measured every square inch of your body, you've marked off time on your calendar, you are all geared up, and you're ready to go. So now what?

Getting motivated to start a program is usually the easiest part. It's the "sticking with it" part that's hard. Knowing how to properly plan your program is an essential aspect of staying with the game plan. In this section, I'll show you safe ways to move forward to avoid burnout. I'll also suggest how to vary your program to prevent boredom. We'll also look at why the beginning and the end of your workout are just as important as the middle, and how stretching and weight training helps. Finally, I'll show you ways to modify your program if needed, as well as sample programs for the beginner and the more experienced walker.

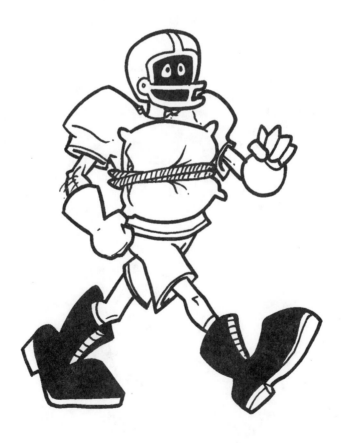

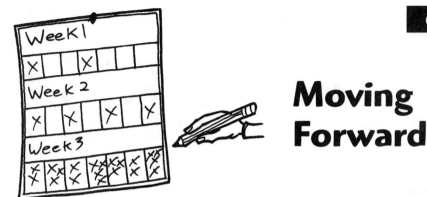

Chapter 5

Moving Forward

In This Chapter

➤ Walking three days a week is good for your health

➤ Start slow to avoid injury and burnout

➤ Is walking alone safe?

➤ Get out of the rut of routine routes

Now that you've gotten all your body parts measured and your walking gear together, you can't wait to get out there and go. Deciding to make a commitment and begin a program can be very exciting. Yet now that you've started, you must learn how to proceed so as not to jeopardize all of your hard work. One of the biggest reasons why people drop out of their exercise routines is because they overdo it. Over-training can cause injury, irritability, insomnia, weight gain or loss, and even depression. Many people, including professional athletes, over-train for fear of losing motivation and fitness. To avoid having this happen to you, I've summarized some guidelines that will help you progress safely. Remember that moderation and balance are the keys here.

Frequency: How Many Days a Week Is Enough?

For beginners, or those of you who scored below average on the fitness tests, the American College of Sports Medicine recommends starting out walking three days a week, which is the minimum requirement to achieve most of the health benefits associated with exercise. ACSM also suggests spreading the days out to avoid working out two days in a row, in order to enable your body to rest and recover on the "off" days.

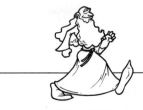

Wise Walkers

Always err on the side of less rather than more. Feeling apathetic about your physical state can be a sign of fatigue.

Walkers Watch Out!

Don't push yourself beyond your physical abilities. If you've scheduled a six-day walking week, but feel tired and over-trained by day four, take a break. Your brain may be scheduling your week, but it's your body that is doing all the work. Listen to it.

Remember that these are general guidelines and do not take into consideration those of you who have medical conditions. If your doctor recommended that you walk only two days a week, then you should stick with this and not try to push it.

If you have been walking for a while, and scored average to above average on most of the fitness tests, then you may increase the number of days per week you walk to four, five, or six. Individuals whose goal is to lose weight may also increase their walking frequency to five or six days a week. Remember: The more you move, the more energy you'll burn and the more weight you will lose. You can also choose to walk every day, but then you should alternate the intensity of your walk from one day to the next. Walking hard and strong every day will eventually wear your body down and cause injury and increase your chances of dropping out of your walking program altogether. If, for example, your walk on Tuesday is an hour-long hill walk, make Wednesday's mild by keeping it slow and flat.

Interesting Facts About Intensity

Intensity refers to the amount of work your body is doing, measured by the speed of your heart rate. As I referred to in Chapter 2, "One Step at a Time," in order to increase your fitness level, you need to stress your cardiovascular system by pushing your heart and muscles to work more than they are accustomed to working. Again, this must be done slowly so as not to overstress the body.

No one formula fits for everyone. Levels of intensity depend on fitness levels, age, health status, and goals. Similarly, different people respond differently to the same stress, and therefore you must pay close attention to how you are feeling as you apply these guidelines to your own program.

In order to prescribe intensity, we must first know how to determine it. In Chapter 2, I discussed your heart rate and three ways to measure intensity during a workout: the Talk Test, palpation, and the heart-rate monitor.

The Talk Test is a way to determine how hard you are working by using your breath and ability to talk. If, while you are walking, you can carry on a conversation without noticing that you need a breath, you are most likely not working your heart too much. If, on the other hand, you can't even get the words out to tell your walking partner to slow down, chances are you are working too hard. Generally, you want to be able to walk and talk—with some effort. Feeling that you need to slow down or to wait until you get to the top of the hill to finish your sentence is okay. On the other hand, if "Madame Butterfly" is flowing freely from your lips, you will probably want to pick it up a bit.

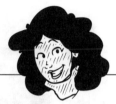

Interesting Excerpts

The Talk Test is synonymous with the Rate of Perceived Exertion method (or RPE) created by a physiologist in 1987. Perceived exertion is the overall distress of your body during exercise. It is a subjective test designed to reflect your own assessment of how hard you think you are working by using a numerical scale where 0 is low effort and 10 is high. As the intensity of your workout increase the level of discomfort and difficulty of breathing also increase. The numerical scale allows you to give subjective evidence of your effort level.

The second way to measure your heart rate is by counting your pulse. In the middle of your workout, during the high-endurance part, place your index finger and your middle finger just below the jaw line to the side of the throat. Chances are, if you are working at all, you will pick it up quite easily. If you can count and walk at the same time, great! If not, stop for a moment, find the rhythm, and count for 15 seconds. Multiply the number by four. Generally speaking, your heart rate should be between 65 and 85 percent of your predicted maximal heart rate (220 – your age). For example, if my maximal heart rate is 180, my heart rate should be somewhere between 120 and 150 during the most intense period of exercise; hovering around 135 to 140 would be good.

Use the tip of the middle and index fingers and place them on the side of the neck, just lateral to the throat. Hold there until you've found a pulse, and then count.

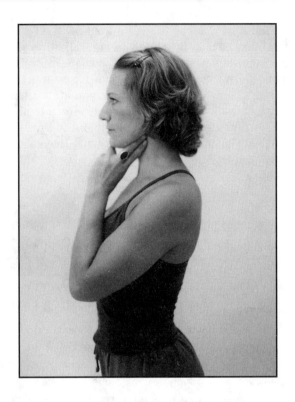

If counting and calculating your pulse seems too complicated and distracting, you can always invest in a heart-rate monitor. These nifty little devices have a strap that wraps around your chest and transmits electromagnetic waves (your heart beat) to a watch-like monitor you attach to your wrist. This way, all you have to do is glance at the monitor to check your heart rate. You pay for the efficiency, however. Heart-rate monitors start at $50 and can get up to $300. Now that you know how to read your heart rate, what's next? Because you are working your body at higher levels than you are used to, you must do it with caution. If you are only working out three days a week, then it is not advised to work at 85 percent of your heart-rate max all three days. A good rule would be to add one day of harder walking for every two days of easy walking (this includes days where you do not walk at all, or "rest days"). Or, to put it a different way, give yourself two easy days between your hard days. For example, if you are walking three days a week, make one of those days a hard day. If you are walking five days a week, try adding another hard day to your program. Remember, adequate rest (at least two days) in between hard days is key for keeping yourself out of trouble. The following is a sample chart that shows a safe distribution of easy to hard days based on the number of days you walk:

Number of Walking Days	Easy	Hard	M	T	W	TH	F	S	S
3	2	1	E		H			E	
4	2	2	E	H		E		H	
5	3	2	E	H		E	H	E	
6	3	3	E	H	E	H	E	H	

Of course, time plays a big role when considering intensity by the fact that they are interchangeable. For example, on your "hard" days, you needn't walk for as long since you are doing more work per minute. Walking one hour at 65 percent of your maximum heart rate is similar to walking half an hour at 80 percent of your maximum heart rate. Even though it's half the time, you are challenging your cardiovascular system considerably at 80 percent. Similarly, if you are only walking at an intensity of 60 percent of your maximum heart rate, you might want to increase the duration of your walk.

Time: Are We Talking Minutes or Hours Here?

By now, you're probably wondering just how long you'll need to work out each exercise period to achieve your goals. Again, that depends on your goals and on your current fitness level. If your goal is to increase how fast you want to walk, then you should focus on picking up the pace rather than extending the workout. For example, 20 to 40 minutes of *interval* walking, one to two times per week, should be adequate to increase your speed.

If, however, you want to lose weight, you will have to get used to long walks since the more you move, the more energy you'll burn and the more weight you'll lose. If your goal is to improve overall fitness, however, you can strike a balance between time, intensity, and frequency, incorporating long, lower-intensity days with short, high-intensity days.

Walkers Watch Out!

Listen to your body!!! Feelings of chronic fatigue, ongoing soreness, and aches and pains are symptoms of over-training, and your body might be telling you that you need a break.

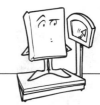

Weighty Words

Interval training involves repetitive sequences of high-intensity exercise bouts with low-intensity active recovery. An example would be walking one loop around a track as fast as you can, followed by walking the second loop at a slower pace, and then repeating this sequence several times.

As I mentioned earlier, there is an important relationship between time and intensity. The higher your intensity, the less time you have to work. Likewise, the lower the intensity, the longer you have to go to reap the same rewards.

The majority of your weekly walking should be moderately long (30 to 40 minutes each session) at a moderate intensity level (65 to 75 percent). As you get stronger, you might want to incorporate a longer, low-intensity walk into your routine—for example, a 40- to 60-minute session at 65 percent MHR. Later, you can add a higher-intensity shorter walk to balance your routine. Give your body adequate rest, even when you don't feel like it. Incorporating "rest" days into your program is crucial to your success as a walker. I will discuss further how to do this in Chapter 9, "Yes! Pain, No Gain."

You can break up your sessions into smaller time frames if doing 20 minutes at a times seems too difficult. If 10 minutes in the morning and 10 minutes in the afternoon is better than 20 minutes all at once, then go ahead and break the time up. Where special needs are concerned, simply moving *more* is the most important thing to remember.

Progressing Patiently

As I mentioned earlier, one of the main reasons why people lose their commitment to exercise is because they do too much too soon. Burn out, injury, and boredom are all negative consequences of trying to work out too much too fast.

Your body needs rest—yes, r-e-s-t—in order to go on. It needs time to adjust to the sudden increase of activity, to replenish energy stores, and to rebuild tissue. Remember, when you exercise, you're putting extra stress on your body, which breaks down tissue and depletes energy stores. In addition, sleep deprivation has been linked to interference with glucose metabolism, and glucose is stored energy. In order to perform adequately next time, your body needs time to repair and to build itself back up. Without rest, your body is in a constant state of depletion and it must "steal" some of the energy you would normally use for your walk to repair and mend itself.

According to the ACSM, you should build up your fitness in three stages. Although somewhat conservative, these stages will help guide you through your program to ensure that you avoid injury and over-training.

The Initial Stage:	4 to 6 weeks
Heart Rate:	40 to 60 percent of HR max
Duration:	15 to 20 minutes
Frequency:	3 times a week

If you've been working out for a while, you may feel this program is a little too easy. Nevertheless, at least try it for a couple of weeks if walking is new to you. Walking works different muscle groups than your former form of exercise, so your body will need time to adjust to the change.

The Improvement Stage:	4 to 5 months
Heart Rate:	50 to 85 percent of HR max
Duration:	Up to 90 minutes
Frequency:	3 to 5 times a week

After your body has adjusted to the initial conditioning stage, it will need to be challenged in order to improve. You need to *overload* it. The improvement stage is a time to push your intensity and your endurance to another level. Generally speaking, you will want to add both time per session and frequency of workouts before you increase intensity. For example, try adding five minutes to your workout every two to three weeks, or adding one to two minutes every week. Or, you might also consider adding a day each month to your routine. You might want to alternate between time and frequency by adding time to each day one month, and adding an extra day per week the next month. Again, be careful not to add too much too soon. In terms of intensity, it all depends on how fit you are and how your body is adjusting to the walking thus far. Again, err on the conservative side. After you've been walking consistently for several months, throw a day of speed-work onto your routine.

Weighty Words

The **overload** principal states that in order for a system to change or adapt, a specific exercise overload that is above normal everyday levels must be applied to the system. This overload, when applied, will help improve fitness in the muscles being worked.

The Maintenance Stage:	After 6 months
Heart Rate:	70 to 85 percent
Duration:	30 to 60 minutes
Frequency:	3 times a week

The maintenance stage, a.k.a. "cruise control," is the minimum amount of exercise you'll need to maintain your fitness once you've gotten past the improvement stage. As I mentioned earlier, these are very general guidelines to help people, mainly beginners, structure their walking routines. In Chapter 10, "In the Beginning," I'll give you more details, including sample programs, so that you can create a routine more specific to your current fitness level and your goals.

The Where, What, Why, and How of Walking

It is a good idea to be prepared when designing your walking program. It helps to minimize disappointment and frustration, which lead to dropping out. Research your neighborhood well, and try to locate city parks and good walking routes. Keep track of your distance and time, which may help keep you motivated. Finally, be prepared to change your program. Variety is key to keeping you interested and challenged. It also helps you avoid injuries associated with repetitive motion.

Avoiding Routine Routes

Map out several routes to explore over the next several weeks. Include a list of all the city parks, lakes, and other recreational areas. Look for sights to see, such as local monuments and historical geography. Make it interesting and fun. Get to know your city. If you are just taking a walk around the neighborhood, choose different streets to walk on. Planning your routes ahead of time will help to keep you focused and will add an element of surprise and adventure to your program.

Keeping Track of Time and Distance

As I mentioned earlier, keeping track of your progress can be very motivating. It'll tell you both how far you've come and how far you still have to go. Some bookstores and many athletic stores sell what is known as training logs. These are spiral-bound notebooks that keep track of your progress. Make sure you choose a *walking* log, as it will provide information specific only to walking. These logs range in their detail and can seem quite complicated at times. Choose a simple one for starters, one that tracks your distance, time, and heart rate. Make sure there's space for notes about a variety of things (e.g., "felt very strong today, breathing easier" or "left ankle pain with hills"). That way you'll be able to look back to your turning points or setbacks and see what may have contributed to either.

You might also consider buying a digital stopwatch. Then you'll be able to know exactly how long you've walked. For people whose goal is to increase speed, you should definitely invest in a watch that clocks the precise time. However small it may seem, shaving a few minutes and even seconds off your time can be very inspiring.

Staying Vitalized by Adding Variety

Finally, change your routine on a regular basis! Boredom is a killer and can increase your chances of dropping from your program entirely. Try not to do the same route every time, as it is sure to get old and boring. You can even mix your routine within the day. You might want to alternate walking one block fast with walking one block slow, for example. Use your imagination and be careful not to get stuck in a rut.

Varying your program has physiological benefits, too. The National Academy of Sports Medicine asserts that by changing your program every three to four weeks, you challenge your body, which helps to prevent plateaus and stagnation.

60

Safety Tips to Consider

Finally, and most important, you must consider your safety while designing your walking program. Walking is an enjoyable activity that temporarily frees you from your everyday routine. It is nice to be able to go out for a walk and let go of everything and to have a few moments of peace. While you do this, however, you must also be cautious of your surroundings.

The following are some guidelines you might want to consider before walking out your door.

Walking Alone

If you can, walk with someone else, particularly at night. It's just safer. Someone is less likely to attack two people than one. If, on the other hand, you cannot or do not want to walk with someone, please take the following factors into consideration:

In the city:

➤ Be aware of your surroundings. Scan the area at all times, and take note of anything unusual.

➤ Walk with purpose and strength in your stride. Walk as if you are going somewhere. You are less of a target for attack when you move with confidence.

➤ Walk in busier areas where there are more people around. Avoid dark secluded streets.

➤ Walk without headphones. Even though this is a hard one to stick to, wearing headphones cuts you off from what is going on around you, making you an easier target.

➤ Walk during the day. If you must walk at night, wear reflective clothing (I will discuss this in more detail later on).

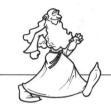

Wise Walkers

Interval training is an excellent way to add variety to your walking routine. Mixing up periods of high and low intensity (walking fast, walking slow) is a great way to push not only your cardiovascular system but your muscular endurance as well.

Walkers Watch Out!

Think about the area you live in. How safe is it? Most police stations can print out a sheet with weekly crime reports per designated area. You might want to check out this sheet to avoid those areas that are heavier in crime incidents.

In the woods:

➤ Walk in daylight.

➤ Map your route ahead of time, and know where you are going.

➤ If you have a cell phone, bring it just in case you do get lost.

➤ Bring a first-aid kit with snakebite instructions.

➤ Know how to avoid wild animals.

➤ Walk with a stick.

Night Walking

Most of us have jobs that limit our walk time to two options: before work and after work. This means that most of the time you will be walking in the dark, which is fine as long as you take the necessary precautions. Fortunately, clothing manufacturers have planned for your busy lives and limited exercise schedules and have created all kinds of reflective gear to keep you visible. Many jackets and shoes have reflective panels sewn onto them. Try to find clothing for your outer layers that have these panels sewn onto the arms, back, and front of your garment. Wear bright clothing. Stay away from grays, blacks, and browns as they blend in with the darkness. White and primary colors catch the eye and are hard to miss. You could always wear fluorescent colors to assure visibility as well.

Defense Do-Dads

There are some little gadgets and tricks you can learn to use to defend yourself in the unlikely event of an attack. They range from hand-held devices to classes and skills learned with practice. Again, I hate to promote fear, but crime is a reality most of us must accept, and the more prepared you are, the less likely you will become a victim.

Pepper spray and mace are now made with a holster, which you can attach to your key chain. Read the instructions carefully to avoid hurting yourself. In fact, you should take a class at a local police station or a YWCA to become accustomed to their use and also to receive certification to carry them, which a few states require. Whistles are another good defense against being attacked. When blown in the ear of someone, serious damage can be done to the eardrum, distracting your attacker from his or her pursuit, therefore giving you a chance to get away. Attach the whistle to your key chain. Wearing it around your neck can be more dangerous than safe, as in the case with the sprays, and can be used against you if you are not careful.

Self-defense classes, however, are probably your best bet to protect yourself against crime. They are usually offered in a variety of places, including the gym, schools, and private studios. Check out your local phone book or community center.

The Least You Need to Know

➤ Walking three days a week for 30 minutes will improve your health.

➤ If you walk at a high intensity, you do not have to walk as long, and vice versa.

➤ Progressing slowly decreases your chances of injury and dropping out.

➤ Plan your routes ahead of time and change them regularly to avoid boredom.

➤ Take precautions to keep yourself safe.

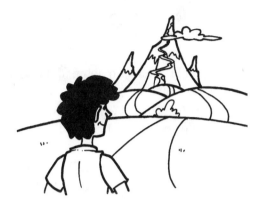

Chapter 6

Now That You've Got the Basics, Let's Have Some Fun!

In This Chapter

➤ Walking hills to burn more calories

➤ How variety keeps you going

➤ Walking with weights to build upper-body strength

➤ From meters to trees, tips for interval training

You started your walking program two months ago. So far you've been really diligent. This past week, however, something seems to have changed. Your walks have become easier and you are not losing any more weight. In addition, you are starting to feel a little bored with your usual route. You want to keep walking, but feel less motivated than you did in the beginning. You'd like to change *something* but you just don't know what. You've reached a plateau in your program. Not to worry. Your body just needs a change, needs a challenge, and that's what this chapter will help you design. I'll show you how to add some weights to your exercise routine, vary the pace, and other change-ups to help you stay interested and motivated.

Turning the Heat up with Hills

Just the thought of climbing up one fills your heart with dread. But before you run and hide, why don't you contemplate the following reasons why you should consider making friends with the mountain: With just a slight incline, you will be burning more calories with each step. The steeper the hill, the more calories you burn.

Walking a hill increases the intensity of your walk, which means you won't have to walk as far to burn the same amount of calories. Just carrying your body weight up the darn thing is intense enough!

Walking up hills works different muscles than walking on flat surfaces. Your front thigh muscles and rear end get a much more concentrated workout as you lift your body up and push it forward. Here are a few safety issues to consider when walking up and down hills:

➤ Keep your body perpendicular to the surface. If you lean forward going up hills or backward as you descend, you'll put too much pressure on your lower back.

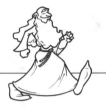

➤ Land on your heel like you do when you walk on flat surfaces, and try to land lightly to avoid jarring your joints.

➤ Take small steps rather than big ones. The leg is already working harder to lift and propel your body forward, and adding length to your stride can be too much for the muscles to handle at first.

➤ Finally, take a little extra time to stretch and warm up the calves. As you walk on uneven surfaces, your ankles and lower legs work extra hard to maintain the stability and balance of the rest of your body. These little muscles need a little extra care, both before and after your hill walk, to prevent injuries such as shin splints and ankle sprains.

Wise Walkers

Turn it up! Increasing the intensity of your walks enables you to get more done in less time, and it increases your cardiovascular endurance and heart strength at a much faster pace while giving you a sense of challenge to prevent boredom.

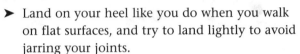

Walkers Watch Out!

If you have had a history of back pain, surgery, or injuries, I recommend that you speak with your doctor before you add hills to your program. Because of the slant, added stress is put on the lower back and can exacerbate problems.

Stepp'n on Stairs

Walking up and down bleachers and steps are another good way to increase the intensity of your workout. In addition to adding some challenge, stair-stepping is a great workout for your rear end, too. Try including a day of bleachers or stairs to add a little variety and intensity to your program.

When walking up stairs, please take the following precautions:

➤ Place your entire foot on the stair. Many injuries are due to careless foot placement.

➤ Make sure you take your time and watch your step (oops, no pun intended ... well, maybe a little).

➤ Lift through the entire leg and push down through the heel, not the ball of your foot. Putting excess stress on the front of your foot can put added stress on your knees and might eventually cause pain or injury.

➤ Keep your stomach firm and tight and your posture upright to support your spine.

Start with two sets of 20 to 40 stairs for now. As you get stronger and build your endurance, you can add a set every other week, depending on how your body feels.

Beach Bum

Beach bum is right: Walking on the beach will help shape up your buttocks fast because your feet sink below the surface and you have to push harder to lift yourself up and out of the sand. You get a better upper-body workout, too, because you'll be pumping your arms more in an attempt both to generate some momentum and to keep your balance. Your lower legs can get super strong walking in the sand as well. Pushing off against a giving surface can be quite a workout for your calves and feet.

As you can imagine, walking on dry sand is a lot more difficult than walking on the wet sand at the water's edge. Dry sand gives a lot more, so your foot ends up sinking a lot deeper, and pushing off takes much more energy. If you do walk on dry sand, do it in spurts. Try walking five minutes at a time and make sure you give yourself enough time to stretch and warm up beforehand. (I discuss some good leg stretches you can do in the next chapter.) Also, it is a good idea to wear shoes when walking in dry sand to avoid cutting yourself on glass, shells, or sharp sticks.

Finally, go prepared! Grab your daypack and fill 'er up. Water is crucial since you will probably be working harder and sweating more than you normally do on concrete surfaces. Continue to replenish your fluids throughout your walk. Also, don't forget to protect your eyes! The sun's glare, especially against the water, can be very intense and dangerous. Never stare directly at its reflection, as this can cause temporary spots in your vision or even damage your eyes. Invest in some good sunglasses that protect your eyes from ultraviolet rays. A hat might be a good addition to ensure protection from the sun for both your eyes and your face. Finally, grab a swimsuit; chances are you'll need it by the time you finish.

Walkers Watch Out!

If you have a history of ankle injury or weak ankles, take extra care when walking on the sand. Even though walking on uneven surfaces can strengthen the joint, it can also lead to injury. Start out by walking on the wet sand first if your ankles are unstable, and do ankle-strengthening exercises in between.

Tromping on Trails

Even though hiking and trail walking are terms that many use interchangeably, I would like to differentiate between the two. When I think of hiking, I think of long periods of time out in the wilderness with trails that are sometimes not so obvious to the naked eye. I think of boots and thick socks. I think of climbing over rocks and jumping over streams: ya know, gett'n down and dirty. My vision of a hike usually involves a knapsack with a blanket and lots of tasty snacks. An "entire day" kind of thing, map and all.

Trail walking, on the other hand, is much less involved. Even though you are out in nature, you can easily see the trail neatly carved out in front of you. Not only has the ground been smoothed out for you but also little signs are posted everywhere, telling you which way to go and where the nearest port-a-potty is. You can wear your regular walking shoes and gear on trails, since chances of your climbing mountains and swinging from tree branches are slim. A trail is much like a hike, but more manicured and conservative.

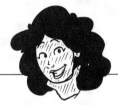

Interesting Excerpts

Most cities have preserved an area of wilderness to be enjoyed by wild and tame mammals (you and me) alike. There are two types of trails: those that loop (one big circle) and those that go out and come back. Some of the mileage is calculated for the entire route and some for half the route (in the case of out and back). Trails range in distance and level of difficulty. The Appalachian Trail, for example, is over 2,000 miles long and stretches from Atlanta all the way up to Maine.

Bring along a small daypack. Even though you might only be gone for an hour or two, it will be useful. Besides your keys, you will need to put several things inside, including a first-aid package with bug repellent, Band-Aids, and a snakebite kit, for starters. Sunscreen and water are two other important items you'll want to throw into your pack. Finally, if you have one, consider taking your cell phone with you. In the unlikely event that you do lose your way, a phone can be a very precious resource to let other people know where you are.

Weights, Anyone?

Walking with weights can benefit you in a few ways. First, dumbbells and ankle weights help work your upper body and legs while adding some variety to your walking routine. Second, your muscles will have to work harder to move you forward, which will burn more calories. Finally, it builds your *stabilizer muscles,* while heightening your sense of balance and perception. I will not be going into detail about weight/strength training until Chapter 8, "Why Weight?"—that's where you'll find specific tips about technique. My focus here is to give you some ideas of how to make your workout a little harder *and* a little more interesting.

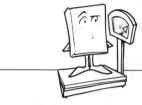

Weighty Words

Stabilizers are those muscles in the front and back of your torso that support (stabilize) the spine. Your stomach and back are categorized as stabilizers, for example.

Your arms play a pretty big role in the efficiency and ease of your gait. Not only do they help to propel you forward but they keep you balanced and in line as well. When you add weights, you can increase the intensity of your workout without having to pick up your speed. Not only are you carrying some additional weight (and therefore burning more calories), but you will also get a more concentrated upper-body workout. Walking with weights also keeps your mind focused on your workout, since you constantly have to count intervals and adjust hand and arm positions. Finally, it is a good way to break up the time by giving you small challenges to keep you occupied along the way.

Hand weights come in a variety of shapes and sizes. Some kinds strap around your wrist, leaving your hands free for water bottles, a dog leash, or keys. You can also buy a pair of lightweight dumbbells, which are good for strengthening not only your arms, but your hands as well. Either type is adequate. You might want to try both to see which one feels more comfortable for you.

Start with one- to two-pound hand weights, even if you are an avid weight lifter. By starting light, you'll allow your body to adapt to the added stress slowly, minimizing your risk of muscle tears and misaligned joints. The following is a list of guidelines that will help to protect you from getting hurt:

➤ Keep your arms close to your body.

➤ Your elbows should be at a 90-degree angle, with your arms at the side of your body.

➤ Make sure that your swing is controlled but not rigid; you want your arms to move in their normal fashion.

➤ Carry a backpack with you to put the weights in, just in case your arms get tired.

➤ Start off your walk with a 10-minute warm-up. While you are walking, warm up your arms by rotating them forward and backward.

69

Once you're warmed up and you've got your weights in hand, you can start out by just swinging your arms gently. Get used to the feel of the weights. When you feel comfortable, you can play with the position of your hands. Notice how, when you turn your palms up, you focus more on the biceps and the chest, but when you turn your palms to face your body, you feel it more in the front and back of your shoulders. On the other hand (no, not literally), extending your arm so it is relatively straight will work your triceps and the side of your back. Again, be gentle. Control the movement and keep your arms close to your body. Walk for 5 minutes using the weights, and then put them in your backpack and walk 10 minutes without them. Repeat this cycle throughout your workout. Add a couple minutes every few weeks until you are walking with weights for the entirety of your walk.

Once you've got the swing of things (couldn't help myself there), try adding a little variety to your walking with weights workout. Add some lateral, front, and back shoulder raises (see Chapter 8 for more information.) Try not to raise your hands above shoulder level, and control, rather than swing, the movement. You could also add a few shoulder presses or shoulder shrugs, or even some bicep curls and tricep kickbacks.

I suggest doing two or three sets of each exercise for 20 to 30 repetitions, making sure you rest in between. If your arms feel tired, put the weights in the backpack and walk without them for a while. Shake out your arms and loosen them up. When you're ready, grab the weight and start again.

Hand and wrist weights are not the only way to add variety and increase the intensity of your workout. Special athletic stores also sell weighted vests, which come with adjustable weight pockets. By increasing the amount of weight you are carrying, you are not only burning more calories, you are also increasing the overall strength and endurance of your muscles.

Walkers Watch Out!

Good form and posture are essential when walking with weights. It is imperative that you not only maintain a controlled swing throughout your workout, but that you also keep your stomach tight and your back upright and strong. Do not walk with weights more than one or two days a week. The purpose here is to add a little variety and to increase the intensity slightly; overdoing it can cause injury and burnout, so keep it simple.

Unfortunately, these vests can get pretty costly. If you do not want to spend the money, you could always buy a pair of 5- to 10-pound ankle weights, and either strap them around your waist or put them in a backpack to carry with you. You will be achieving the same results for a lot less money.

You will notice that, by adding only a few extra pounds, your equilibrium might be a little shaky at first. This is not unusual. You have probably become quite used to how your body feels in space. When you suddenly add weights to the picture, it takes a while for your body and mind to adjust to the change. It is during this adjustment phase when your stabilizers are put to work as they struggle to regulate your gait.

Breaking Up the Time: Fartlek and Interval Training

Another great way to add variety while increasing the intensity of your walks is to interval train, which involves combining lower-intensity with higher-intensity periods of exercise within the same workout. Interval training helps to push your fitness to a different level. It also increases caloric expenditure and tolerance to muscle fatigue so you can walk stronger and longer with more ease. Finally, it adds some variety to your routine to keep your mind and your body challenged and distracted from boredom.

So, how fast should you walk during these "higher-intensity periods"? Well, that all depends on your fitness level. The more experienced a walker you are, the faster you can go. However, if you're just beginning, or have never really pushed your pace, you'll want to start out at a medium pace and work your way up. An example of a beginner's interval would look like this:

1. Warm up for 10 minutes by walking around the track at a slow to medium pace.

2. Set your stopwatch and start your first interval lap; walk at a medium to high pace.

3. Stop your watch when you've completed the lap, and walk around the track at your normal pace.

4. Set your stopwatch and start your second interval lap, walking at a medium to high pace. Try to beat your time by a few seconds.

5. Repeat this sequence for 30 minutes or for 2 miles, whichever comes first.

This is an easy way to introduce yourself to interval training. It is neither too hard nor too easy, and it enables you to challenge yourself with your own pace. Another way to interval train is to pick up the pace on the "straights" of the track and walk slowly in the curves (don't forget to warm up first!). This is a little bit harder than the first workout since you are breaking up the intervals into smaller time increments, thus giving your heart less time to recover. Still another suggestion is to push the pace for half the distance of the track and then walk slower for the other half, and repeat that sequence for two to four miles. Again, this might be better for those of you who have been walking for a while. More advanced walkers might try picking up the pace for two laps around, slowing down for one, picking up for two, and so on....

Walkers Watch Out!

Avoid doing more than one interval day a week in the beginning. Your body will need time to recover, and pushing yourself too much might cause injury, fatigue, and even illness.

You can also measure intervals by heart rate. The best way to do this is to purchase a heart-rate monitor (remember those funny things you strap around your chest?). Calculate your predicted max heart rate (PMHR) by subtracting your age from 220. Once you've got this number, you are going to figure a series of four ranges (or zones) based on percentages of your PMHR. Zone 1 should be somewhere between 60 to 65 percent of MHR, zone 2: 65 to 75 percent, zone 3: 75 to 80 percent and zone 4: 80 to 90 percent. Get out your calculator and determine your zones based on your predicted maximal heart rate. For example, to calculate a 45-year-old's predicted max heart rate and his or her 1, 2, 3, and 4 zones you would do the following:

220 – 45 years = 175 (predicted maximal heart rate)

175 × 60 to 65 percent = 105 to 114   Zone 1

175 × 65 to 75 percent = 114 to 130   Zone 2

175 × 75 to 80 percent = 130 to 140   Zone 3

175 × 85 to 90 percent = 148 to 157   Zone 4

During your regular walks you want to keep your heart rate between zones 1 and 2, occasionally raising it to level 3. On interval-training day, however, you should work your heart in zone 2, but mostly 3, and occasionally 4. Once your heart rate is up in level 3, you will want to keep it there for anywhere between 30 seconds and 90 seconds. Here is a sample program using the example in the preceding table.

Minute	Zone	Heart Rate
1 to 10	1	105 to 114
10 to 14	2	114 to 130
15	3	130 to 140
16	2	114 to 130
17 to 18	3	130 to 140
19	2	114 to 130

Minute	Zone	Heart Rate
20 to 21	3	130 to 140
22	2	114 to 130
23 to 24	3	130 to 140
25 to 34	2	114 to 130
35 to 40	1	105 to 114

If you haven't got 40 minutes to walk, or if you'd like to walk for longer than 40 minutes, you can subtract or add intervals to accommodate your time schedule. Just remember not to skip out on your warm-up or cool-down. I will explain why in the next chapter.

As you can see, you have many ways to keep your walking workout interesting. All you need is a little imagination (and a lot of red cars!). Remember to take it slow. Allow your body time to adjust to the added stress. Pay attention to how you feel. If you are tired and unmotivated, take a day off. If you feel like you are pushing yourself too hard, slow down. Don't sacrifice your health for your program. Of course, if you prefer not to change your routine, don't. If mixing things up is too confusing and overwhelming, stick with what you have been doing. The most important thing to do is to keep moving.

The Least You Need to Know

➤ Hills increase the intensity of your walk without having to increase speed.

➤ Walking in the sand is harder because it has less stability to push off against.

➤ Hiking and trail walking are two separate activities.

➤ Walking with weight increases the number of calories you burn while increasing your strength.

➤ Interval training is a good way to challenge your body while occupying your mind.

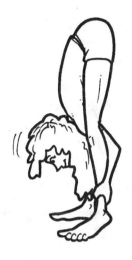

Chapter 7

Warming Up, Cooling Down, and Yes! Stretching

In This Chapter

➤ Waking up to warming up

➤ Why cooling down counts

➤ Staying flexible to keep you safe from injury

➤ Sample stretches for starting out

You've barely carved enough time into your schedule for your weekly walks, and now I'm going to ask you to do what? To stretch? Who has time to stretch, let alone warm up and cool down? But warming up, cooling down, and stretching are the most important aspects of your walking program. They help to prepare your body for the battle, keep you free of injury, maximize your performance, eliminate waste products from your system, and ease you back down into slow-mo. In this chapter, I'll show you how to prepare your body for, and recover from, exercise.

The Importance of a Warmed–Up Walker

Not giving yourself enough time to warm up can result in cramping, overheating, and serious injury. Warming up enables your muscles and your heart to adjust comfortably to the increase of energy suddenly being demanded of them. A proper warm-up will increase blood flow to the working muscles while loosening up the joints and connective tissues. It will also slowly raise your body temperature to prevent you from overheating and passing out.

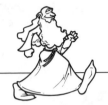

Wise Walkers

The purpose of a warm-up is to gradually increase your heart rate, blood pressure, oxygen consumption, and dilation of blood vessels, as well as the heat and elasticity of your active muscles.

You should spend at least 5 to 10 minutes warming up before you begin your workout. Most experts agree that simulating your workout, but at a slower pace, is adequate. You could, for example, start your walk at 50 percent of your normal workout pace and then, after 5 minutes, pick it up to 75 percent; then when you've hit 10 minutes, start walking at your usual workout level. Be sure to listen to your body. If you don't feel adequately warmed up after 10 minutes, add an extra 5. You'll know you're warmed up when your body temperature rises, your breathing is a little heavier, your heart rate has picked up slightly, and your muscles feel looser.

Doing some warm-up exercises at home before you go out for your walk would be okay, too. The following is a list of a few tricks that would work to warm up your walking muscles before you step out the door:

➤ March in place for five minutes. Lunge side to side for five minutes.

➤ Walk up and down the stairs 5 to 10 times.

➤ Sit down on a chair (sofa, bed ...) and stand up. Repeat 10 times. Rest. Do three sets.

March in place at a regular pace. Once you feel your heart stimulated, lift your knees higher so that they are parallel with the floor. Repeat for 5 to 10 minutes.

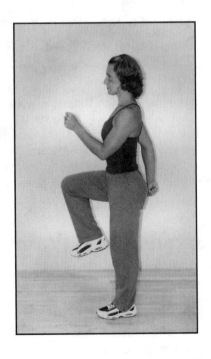

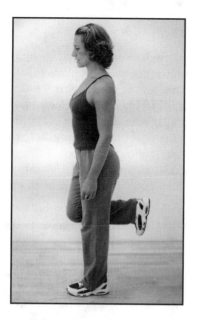

March in place at a regular pace. Once you feel your heart stimulated, lift your feet back behind you so that your calf is parallel with the floor. Repeat for 5 to 10 minutes.

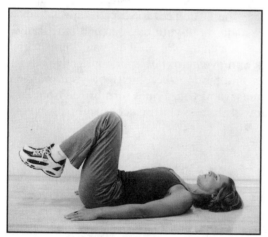

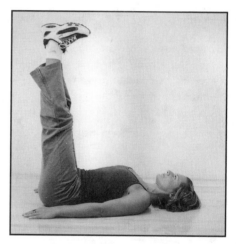

Lie on the floor on your back. With your legs together, lift your feet off the floor. Straighten and bend your legs 10 times.

I suggest varying your warm-up just to see what works best for you. Keep it challenging and fun so you will look forward to it. If you are pressed for time, do not skip the warm-up. Shorten it to five minutes, but make sure that you feel warmed up when you begin to walk and that you are not just going through the motions.

The Cool Cat Cool-Down

During exercise, your body has been challenged and stimulated. Blood flow, body temperature, and chemical combustion have been taking place for the past 20, 30, or 40 minutes. Your body has found a rhythm and is going with the flow, and you want to just stop suddenly? Cooling down brings the heart rate down slowly. It redistributes the blood and oxygen from the working muscles to the brain. It removes waste products such as *lactic acid* and carbon dioxide from your muscles and lungs and basically just teases you back into slow motion, giving your body a chance to readjust its energy systems. A proper cool-down should last from five to 10 minutes and should be the reverse of your warm up. Again, take your time. Remember, your body knows best. So listen to it!

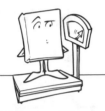

Weighty Words

Lactic acid is the waste product left in your tissues during and after exercise. Inadequate oxygen in the muscles may cause this build-up.

Why Stretch?

When I ask clients how much time they spend stretching, nine out of 10 of them will look away and mumble something that sounds like "not enough," which usually, in my experience, translates into "none." Well, guess what? You *need* to stretch, especially if you spend the majority of your day perched practically motionless in a chair. Not only do your joints stiffen from lack of movement, but your connective tissues, ligaments, and tendons become tight, your muscles become tense, and your bones turn brittle from lack of use. You begin to feel little aches and pains everywhere.

Perfecting Posture

Stretching helps to realign any imbalance of your *soft tissues*. Muscle imbalances develop as the stronger muscles try to compensate for the weaker ones. This, of course, puts more pressure not only on the muscle, but on the joint as well, sometimes causing the joint to be pulled or pushed out of alignment. If you maintain a consistent stretching regimen, however, you are helping to decrease the tension of the tighter muscles. With the reduction of muscle tension and tightness, you automatically improve your posture. Your joints feel less stiff and you begin to stand (and walk) taller.

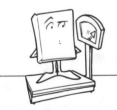

Weighty Words

Soft tissue refers to—among other things—your muscles, ligaments, and tendons.

Daily Doings

Even everyday tasks, such as picking things up off the floor, reaching for the can of soup on the top shelf, or securing your child into the car seat, can be quite taxing on your muscles and joints when your muscles aren't strong and pliable. Sudden movement, or even extending yourself, can cause damage to the ligaments and tendons as well. When your muscles are supple from stretching, they give more to the pressure that is being exerted on them, decreasing your risk of sprains, strains, and other injuries.

Joint Ventures

Finally, stretching allows more flexibility and *range of motion* (*ROM*) in the joint. Greater ROM means more movement. With more movement, you have an increase of nutrition moving in and waste products moving out of the joint structure. They will become more lubricated and less stiff, and will begin to feel more stable, supportive, and strong.

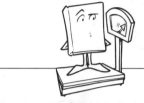

Weighty Words

ROM, or **range of motion,** refers to the amount of motion allowed between two bony levers.

How Often and How Much?

So, I've managed to convince you to include stretching in your program. Now what? You have heard so many conflicting views on the "do's" and "don'ts" of stretching that you don't know what or whom to believe. Is it 20 minutes or 20 seconds? Do you bounce or do you hold? Should you stretch before or after you work out? So many questions! I know it's confusing, but that's okay because I'm here to help.

How?

You can stretch in several ways, but for the sake of simplicity, I am only going to mention a couple. First, you can try the static stretch. Static refers to no motion. When you stretch a muscle using the static approach, you stretch a muscle to the point of slight discomfort and hold the position for 10 to 30 seconds, repeating the sequence two or three times.

Second, there is the dynamic or active stretch, which does involve movement. Swinging your arms, lunging from side to side, and twisting your torso can all be categorized as dynamic stretches. You must be careful with dynamic stretches, however. If your muscles are not warmed up and you start swinging them, you could do some damage to the connective tissue and muscles around the joints. Take it easy and start out slow. And always make sure that you are adequately warmed up!

Coming Equipped

Believe it or not, you can use many tools to help you stretch, including big green balls, ropes, rubber tubing, towels, and other people, to name just a few. Although it's not required, using equipment to stretch can be handy.

First, it helps you reach those places on your body that are too far away to grab with your hand. Take the supine hamstring stretch, for example. In this exercise, you lie on your back with one leg extended, and then grab your foot and pull it down toward your body. Yeah, right. Only superheroes like Elastic Man can do stuff like that. Normal people like you and me, however, can use a towel, a rope, or a rubber tube to do the trick. Just wrap it around the flat part of your foot and gently pull your leg toward your body.

Lie on your back with your feet on the floor and your knees bent. Lift one leg up so that it is straight over your body, and wrap a towel around the ball and the arch of your foot. Gently pull the foot toward your head. Bend the knee slightly if needed. Hold for 10 to 20 seconds and release.

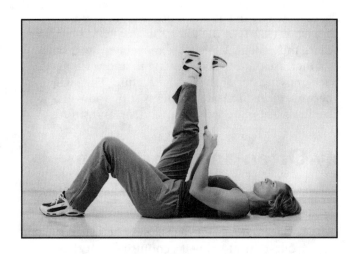

Second, tools can add a greater range of motion to deepen and intensify your stretch. I love the "green ball" for this kind of stretch. The green ball (or therapy ball) was originally designed to help physical therapy patients rehabilitate and strengthen injured limbs. Because of their incredible effectiveness, however, many gyms have purchased these balls to be used by their regular members.

You can purchase a therapy ball at back- and spine-care facilities, or online if you search under "physioball" or "therapy ball." Many come with a video, which I suggest you review before tackling any of the exercises. No matter what position I'm in, I always feel a greater range of motion due to the height and curvature of the ball. I can stretch further and in more positions than when I'm lying or sitting on a flat surface.

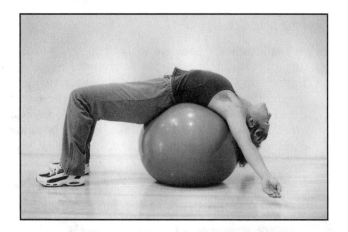

First, have a seat on the ball. Once you feel stable, roll down along your spine until your entire back is on the ball. Slowly lie back, letting your arms fall out to the sides and your head fall back. Try to relax all of your muscles. If you are doing it right, you should feel an amazing stretch down the entire front of your body.

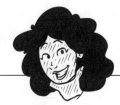

Interesting Excerpts

The "Swiss ball" (a.k.a. physioball) was first introduced in 1963 by an Italian manufacturer by the name of Aquilino Cosani, who designed them initially as toys for children. Swiss balls started being used in other areas of Europe as a means of physical rehabilitation shortly afterward. In fact, 1970 marks the year when the ball was introduced as a rehabilitative device at the World Physical Therapy Congress in Amsterdam by the Swiss doctor Susan Klein-Vogelbach. "Swiss balls" were first introduced to the United States in 1975 by two physical therapists studying in Europe.

How Often

You should take the time to stretch every day if possible. Stretching for 20 minutes every day will greatly improve your overall sense of health and well-being. If you can't manage it every day, make sure that you do so at least every time you exercise, preferably before and after your workout, as long as your muscles are warm. Stretching is particularly effective after your walk. Because you've been moving around for the past 30 minutes or more, your muscles are warm and pliable and it is at this time that you'll want to spend at least 20 minutes stretching.

Walkers Watch Out!

Do not push your stretch past the point of mild discomfort. This could cause damage to your soft tissue, forcing you to quit your walking routine entirely.

How Much

As I said earlier, a good stretching regimen means setting aside some time, at least 20 minutes and preferably 30, after each workout. You should stretch every major muscle in your body, starting with those you used the most. In the case of walking, it would be your legs and back. Hold each stretch, at a level of mild discomfort, for 20 to 30 seconds and then rest for several seconds and repeat.

Sample Stretches for Your Lower and Upper Body

Here are some sample stretches that focus primarily on the muscles you use when you walk. Be sure to follow the directions carefully and make sure that you are warmed up and ready before you proceed.

While standing, grab your hands behind your back and lift them up until you feel a stretch in the front of your shoulders. Be sure to keep your back straight and your shoulders relaxed. Hold for 20 to 30 seconds and release. Repeat two or three times.

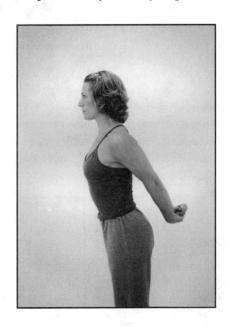

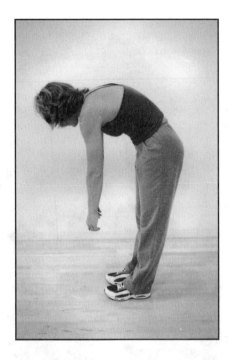

Stand with your feet pointing straight ahead and hips' width apart. Squeeze your buttocks as you slowly lower your torso down, allowing your arms to dangle. Keep your spine rounded and your upper body relaxed. Stop before you start bending at the hips and just hang there for 10 to 20 seconds. Rotate slowly dropping one hand lower than the other. Switch sides.

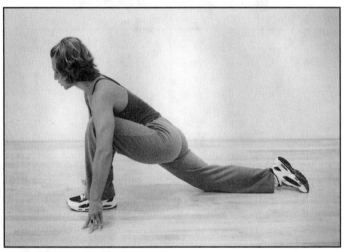

Kneel on the floor and place one foot in front of the body, keeping your knee over your ankle. With the other leg behind you, knee on floor and top of foot facing down, slowly press your hips forward until you feel a stretch. Hold for 20 to 30 seconds and relax. Repeat two or three times and then switch legs.

Grab hold of a chair or stand alongside a wall with your feet hips' width apart. Hold the top of one foot with the opposite hand. Squeeze the buttocks and press the hips forward slightly. Keep the standing leg straight but not locked. Hold for 20 to 30 seconds and relax. Repeat two or three times and then switch legs.

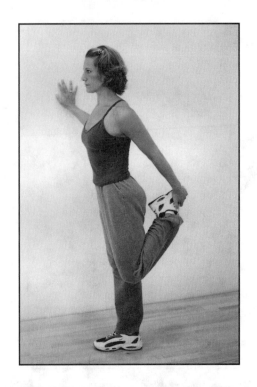

Lie down on your back. Bend both legs, with your feet off the floor. Place the side of the left foot across the right knee so that the left knee rotates externally. Clasp your hands behind the right knee and slowly pull it toward your chest. Hold for 20 to 30 seconds and relax. Repeat two or three times and then switch legs.

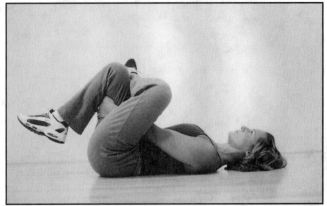

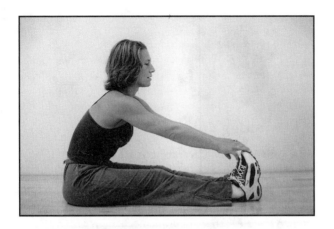

Sit on the floor with your legs straight out in front of you. Flex your feet and keep your back straight as you slowly bend forward at the hip. Imagine touching your chest, not your forehead, to your knees. Ease into this stretch. Do not bounce. Hold for 20 to 30 seconds and relax. Repeat two or three times and then switch legs.

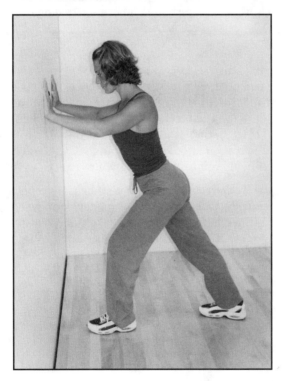

Stand a couple of feet away from a wall or some other support you can put your weight on. Place one leg in front of you, keeping a slight bend at the knee. The other leg should be behind you and straight, with the entire foot on the floor and the toes pointing forward. With your hips in line with the straight leg, slowly lean forward, keeping the back heel planted on the ground. Hold for 20 to 30 seconds and then repeat. Switch legs.

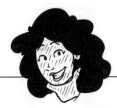

Interesting Excerpts

It is believed that when a muscle is stretched, energy is stored within the fibers. This stored energy becomes available during contraction, which explains why those athletes who stretch more usually perform better. The muscle also has a protective measure built into it so that when it stretches too much, it will automatically contract to keep it from tearing. This is what is known as the "muscle spindle." There is also a mechanism within the muscle that causes it to relax automatically when too much stress is being exerted on it.

As you can see, stretching will take some time. If you really don't have enough time to complete the entire sequence two or three times, just do it once. But make sure you do it! If you really have no time, then try to fit in these stretches throughout the day, while you're sitting at your desk (ankles, neck), standing in the kitchen (lower back, shoulders, chest, sides, and thighs), or getting ready for bed (hamstrings, glutes). Really try to be diligent about your stretches. By doing so, you will be improving your overall sense of well-being, plus minimizing your chances of injury.

Again, make sure that you adequately warm up before you stretch or go out for your walk. Likewise, take the time to slow down before you completely stop walking. Allow the body to adapt slowly to the change in activity. Make sure your heart rate has dropped to its normal level, or just above, before beginning any of these stretches, particularly those that require you to lower your head below your heart.

The Least You Need to Know

➤ Warming up will decrease your chances of injury.

➤ Cooling down transitions your body from higher to lower levels of energy output.

➤ Stretching promotes muscle balance and relaxation, as well as enhancing your performance during everyday activities.

➤ Stretch only when your muscles are warm.

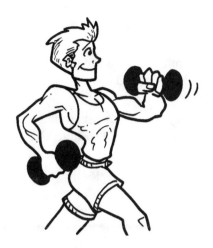

Chapter 8

Why Weight?

In This Chapter

➤ Why weight training works

➤ The difference between free weights and machines

➤ Some alternative strength-training options

➤ Some sample routines to choose from

It may seem strange at first that I have devoted an entire chapter to weight training in a book that is primarily for walkers. But both a weight lifter and a walker need to maintain strong muscles in order to support the bones and joints. Osteoporosis and an attempt to fight bad posture are two other reasons why you might find walkers and weight lifters side by side asking, "You done with those 15-pounders?"

No matter what your exercise preference is, weight lifting is an essential addition to your health regimen. In this chapter, I'll give you some tips to help you develop a safe and effective weight-training regimen.

The Importance of a Strong Body

Aside from the fact that weight training helps to keep your body strong and your joints protected, it also serves several other functions:

➤ **Improved posture.** The stronger your back and stomach muscles are, the taller you stand.

➤ **Increased performance.** Strength builds endurance, and endurance wards off fatigue.

➤ **Healthier bones and joints.** Stressing your muscles pulls on your bones, thereby stimulating more growth and preventing age-related diseases such as osteoporosis and osteoarthritis.

➤ **Decrease in sports-related injuries.** If you build the muscles around the joint, it helps to take some of the weight off the bones and to distribute it to your muscles instead. Muscle tissue is pliable, and helps to absorb and distribute the load of your body weight off your joints, thereby protecting them from fractures and other injuries.

➤ **Revved-up metabolism.** Muscle requires more calories to subsist than does fat or other tissue—it burns more energy even at rest, helping you lose or maintain your weight without as much effort. (See the following table.)

Body Weight	Calories Burned per Minute	Calories Burned per Hour
110 lbs.	5.8	348
120 lbs.	6.5	390
130 lbs.	6.8	408
140 lbs.	7.5	450
150 lbs.	7.9	474
160 lbs.	8.6	516
170 lbs.	8.9	534
180 lbs.	9.6	576
190 lbs.	10.0	600
200 lbs.	10.6	636

These numbers are based on completing a full hour (nonstop) of relatively hard resistance training. Chances are, you will take a break here and there (in fact, it is strongly recommended that you do). If you want to know how many calories you burned during your weight-training session, subtract the minutes of "rest" that you took from the total amount of time you worked out, and multiply this number by calories burned per minute (column two) based on your weight. This will give you a general idea of how many calories you burned during your workout.

How Often and How Much

Have I convinced you yet? I hope so. But before you jump into a rigorous routine of heavy bodybuilding, you should keep some general warnings in mind. First and foremost, you must start slow! Your body needs time to adapt to this new set of demands being put on it. Then, begin using lighter weights. You want to be able to lift a weight at least eight times, but no more than 15, before you feel completely fatigued. If you're having trouble completing eight repetitions, then lower the weight by a few pounds. If, on the other hand, you can lift a weight for endless amounts of time, then you need to increase the weight by several pounds. Start with eight to 15 repetitions. Make sure you are slow with both the contract and release portion of each repetition. When doing a bicep curl, for example, it is a good idea to count two seconds as you lift the weight up and two seconds as you release it. If you find that your form is faltering, then it probably means that your muscles are tired. Take a 30- to 60-second break and then start again. When you feel comfortable, add another set to each exercise.

Begin with one set per *major muscle* group for the first several weeks. Once you feel comfortable, add another set to each exercise. Generally speaking, you need not perform more than three sets per body part per workout.

You should try to take a day off in between workouts. When a muscle fiber has been adequately *overloaded* it means that its fibers have been broken down and it needs at least a day to repair and heal from the "trauma" exerted on it. With sufficient resting time, the muscle will repair stronger than before. If, on the other hand, you do not give your muscles enough time to heal, your body will be in a constant state of repair and the fibers will never have a chance to build strength.

One final thing you should consider when designing your weight-training routine is variety. Your muscles adapt to patterns of repetitive movement so that they eventually become more efficient at performing that movement over time—and your body's natural instinct is to preserve energy. If you don't change your program on a continual basis, your system will get used to the patterns of movement and eventually level off and stop changing. This is what many weight trainers refer to as a *plateau*.

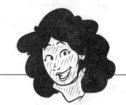

Interesting Excerpts

Did you know that back injuries are not usually the cause of a single incident but are usually due to daily wear-and-tear on the discs of the spine? Ruptured discs are often the straw that broke the camel's back, so to speak.

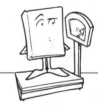

Weighty Words

Strength, endurance, and hypertrophy of a muscle will increase only when the muscle is **overloaded** by working it against loads that are above those it normally encounters.

In order for your muscles to continue developing and growing, you must continue to challenge them. This is why it is important to vary your routine every month or two. By altering the patterns of movement performed during weight training, you'll increase your body's physiological response, thereby stimulating growth and improvement.

The Tools You'll Need

You can increase your strength in many ways. There are, for example, tools like tubing, "Swiss balls," body weight, and free weights that all work perfectly well in building muscle strength and endurance. For the sake of simplicity, however, I am going to stick with free weights since they are probably the most familiar to the vast majority of you.

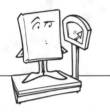

Weighty Words

Plateau refers to a leveling off or an evening out of change, and it is associated with, among other things, cardiovascular, strength, weight-loss, and flexibility programs.

Walkers Watch Out!

Many barbells have screw-like attachments that hold the weights in place. These parts screw on and off easily so you can adjust your weight accordingly. Unfortunately, many people do not check to make sure these end pieces are screwed on tight enough, and they end up with bruised (and sometimes broken) toes due to falling weights.

Free Weights

Free weights refer to weights that are unattached or "free" from a machine. The most common form of free weights includes dumbbells and barbells. Dumbbells differ from barbells in that they are separate entities, so that each limb is challenged individually. Barbells, on the other hand, are operated using two hands so that more than one limb is being used simultaneously. The advantage of using dumbbells over a barbell is that you are better able to determine strength discrepancies from one limb to the next. The weaker "side" cannot freeload with the stronger side and, instead, has to fend for itself.

When you use a barbell, it is not unusual for the stronger side to overcompensate for its weaker counterpart, which inevitably encourages the discrepancy rather than rectifying it. The advantage to using barbells over dumbbells, however, is that you can lift more weight with each repetition. The strength of two limbs rather than one is greater so it's easier to push the limits of your strength a little more by using a barbell. The best solution is to alternate between barbells and dumbbells so that you can catch your weaker spots while pushing your strength to greater capacities.

Everything has its advantages and disadvantages, including free weights. Because free weights are literally "free" from structure, they require a lot more stability and attention to form precision. When using free weights, you must maintain proper body alignment and control of movement or else you risk throwing the rest of your body off and, in the worst case, injuring your back or some other body part. The key with free weights, therefore, is to memorize proper form and to start light. Although this does not ensure an injury-free routine, it does substantially reduce your risk of getting hurt.

Another advantage to using free weights is that you can use them in the comfort of your own home, or anywhere else, for that matter. Equipment is relatively inexpensive as well as easy to adjust, and it can be easily transported if necessary. All you really need is a set of ankle weights and several sets of dumbbells to design a complete weight program. If you can, buy 10-pound ankle weights that have adjustable one- or two-pound weights attached to them so that you can add and remove resistance as needed. The same goes for the dumbbells. Try to buy ones that can be adjusted.

Many sports stores sell adjustable hand weights, which come with a set of plates that can be added and removed with just the twist of a knob. If adjustable weights don't sound appealing to you, you can buy weights that are covered in vinyl or chrome and come in pairs ranging in weight from two to 100 pounds. These are usually a little more expensive since you have to buy them separately, but they work just as well as any other to build your muscles.

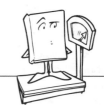

Weighty Words

The **prime-mover** muscles are those muscles that initiate and dominate a movement. For example, the prime mover in an arm curl would be the biceps, while the stabilizing muscles would be the shoulder and forearm muscles.

Machine Madness

The second most popular form of weight training is the machine. Machines serve a different purpose than free weights in two ways. For one, they provide variable resistance throughout a movement. Unlike their free counterparts, which vary in load depending on the angle of resistance, machines have been designed to match the strength curve of a muscle group and its range of motion. This is accomplished by using a system of cables and pulleys, which are organized to distribute the resistance evenly through a range of motion of a particular joint. If you join a gym, ask an instructor to show you the ropes to avoid injury.

A Weight Walker's Wonderland

It is no secret that strengthening your legs, calves, and buttocks is an important part of walking. Because these are the primary muscles (*prime movers*) involved in walking, it is a good idea to make sure that they are prepared for all the stren-uous activity you are about to put them through. A strong lower body will not only reduce your risk of injury, it will also help your overall endurance and power, enabling you to walk longer, faster, and farther.

Walkers Watch Out!

Despite the fact that it is one of the most active joints in the body, the knee is poorly constructed and is therefore a major site for injury and pain.

Upper-body strength is important, too! Whether you are aware of it or not, you are employing the use of your arms, back, chest, and shoulders when you walk as well.

Your arms help to propel you forward as well as keep you in balance. Imagine how difficult it would be to walk if you had your arms tied behind your back? Not easy! Having a strong upper body will definitely assist you in your pursuit to be the perfect walker, so don't ignore them.

When performing any weight training, it is imperative that you maintain good form throughout the exercise. This means that you must concentrate entirely on what you are doing while you are doing it. Keep the motion slow and controlled and don't try to rush through it. Always keep your stomach tight and your torso steady. You must pay close attention to your lower back since this is the area on your body that is at most risk with weight training. If you feel any pain or discomfort, stop and rest. And make sure you *breathe*. Many people make the mistake of concentrating too hard on what they are doing and they forget to breathe.

Wise Walkers

When you breathe, it is important to exhale during the exertion phase of the exercise and to inhale as you release the weight. During a bicep curl, for example, you will exhale as you bend your elbow, and inhale as you straighten it.

Lower-Upper-Body Strengtheners

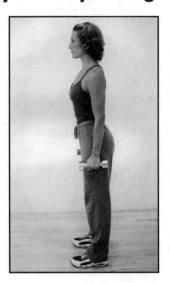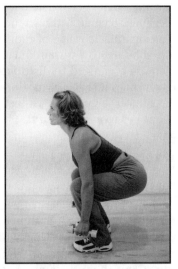

Stand with your feet hips' width apart with your weight in hand by your side. Slowly lower your hips until your knees are at a 90-degree angle, and then lift. Make sure the weight is in your heels and that your stomach is taut. Repeat 10 to 12 times.

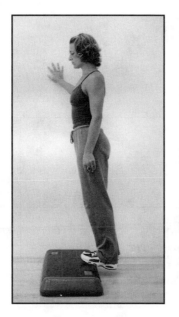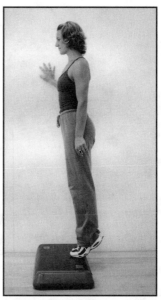

Stand on a step against the wall so you can hold on for support. With your heels off the step, lower your weight until you feel a slight stretch in your calves, and then lift up. Repeat 10 to 12 times.

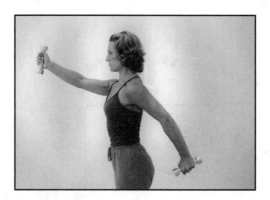

With light weights in hand and with palms facing your body, lift one arm out in front of you to chest level and the other in back of you. Do not twist the shoulders or rotate the hips. Hold for one to three seconds and switch.

93

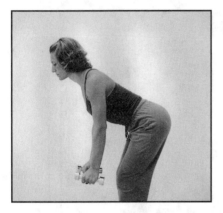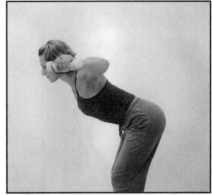

With your weights in hand, bend slightly at the hips. Keep your back straight and your head and shoulders in line. With your arms bent at your sides, lift the dumbbells out to the sides, squeezing the shoulder blades together. Hold for a second and slowly release. Repeat 10 to 12 times.

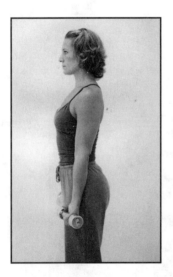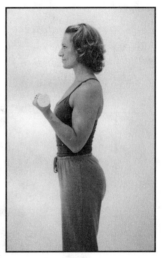

Stand with your feet hips' width apart and your weights in hand, palms facing out. While keeping your elbows glued to your sides, curl the dumbbell until your fists are at shoulder level. Slowly lower and repeat 10 to 12 times.

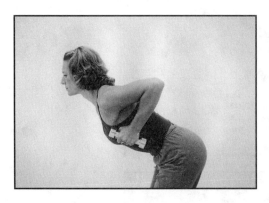 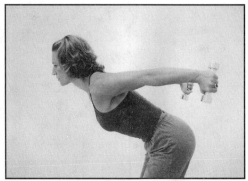

Stand with your feet hips' width apart and your weights in hand, palms facing in toward each other. Bend slightly at the hips and lift the elbows up so that the upper arms are almost parallel with the floor. Extend the arms back, keeping the elbows fixed. Release and repeat 10 to 12 times.

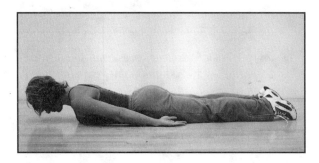

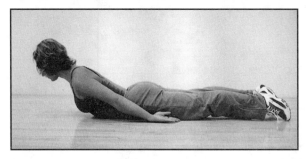

Lie face down with your arms at your sides and your legs together. Keeping your head and shoulders in line, squeeze your buttocks and lift your torso until your chest comes off the floor. Hold for two to five seconds and then slowly release. Repeat 10 to 12 times.

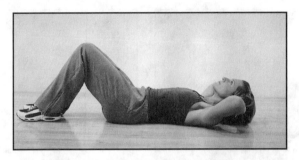

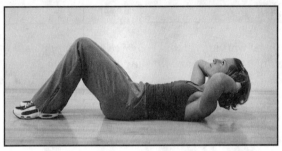

Lie on your back with your knees bent. Clasp your hands behind your head and point your chin toward the ceiling. Pressing your lower back into the floor, lift your shoulder blades off the floor. Hold for one to three seconds and slowly release. Repeat 10 to 20 times.

Walkers Watch Out!

If you have had any problems with your lower back, shoulders, ankles, or knees in the last five years and you feel pain during these exercises, stop doing them and consult your doctor or a physical therapist for modifications.

The Least You Need to Know

➤ Weight training increases bone density.

➤ You can speed up your metabolism by building more muscle.

➤ Breathing correctly is an important part of weight training.

➤ Muscles must be overloaded in order to strengthen.

➤ Resistance exercises are not limited to free weights.

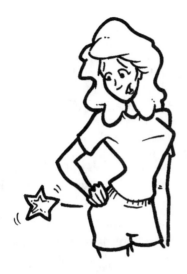

Chapter 9

Yes! Pain, No Gain

> ## In This Chapter
>
> ➤ When and why you should listen to your pain
>
> ➤ Ways to work around boredom
>
> ➤ Danger signs warning you to stop
>
> ➤ Scheduling breaks into your routine
>
> ➤ Walking for lifelong, that's how long

You've probably heard the saying "no pain, no gain." According to my interpretation, the message implies that if you don't hurt then you are not working hard enough to achieve any results. This is simply not true. In fact, pain can be a very important warning signal telling you to slow down or stop exercising entirely.

What many of us don't understand is that our bodies are a lot more in tune than our minds are. If we try too hard, our bodies will know it and will tell us to stop. Injury, illness, excessive and prolonged fatigue, insomnia, and depression are just a few of the by-products of over-training. The same thing is true if you try to exercise while you're sick: Do so, and your body will usually let you know in a big way what a mistake you made.

In this chapter, I will try to answer your questions about the do's and don'ts of exercise. I will also guide you through a safe and healthy approach to exercise so you can continue to walk happily for as long as you are able.

Pondering Pain

There is a very good reason why we have evolved equipped with a biological mechanism in our bodies that perceives pain. Pain warns us of danger. It reminds us of our physical limits and it tells us when we should stop. Without it we'd be in big trouble. But despite this fact, many of us insist on ignoring our pain. In fact, many of us respect and find integrity in moving around, beyond, or despite pain. We believe it builds "character" and makes us stronger, macho, or just plain ambitious. Hard work and overcoming obstacles is a good thing, to a certain extent. We reach a point, however, when we must listen to our bodies or else risk doing long-term and even permanent damage. If we ignore certain types of pain for long enough we can, and will, do irreparable damage and can even risk losing our lives.

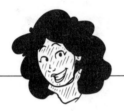

Interesting Excerpts

About 5 to 15 percent of elite athletes may encounter over-training each year, while about 25 to 30 percent experience partial signs of the condition.

Wise Walkers

Over-training is associated with overuse injuries. Overuse injuries are injuries caused by repetitive micro-trauma that leads to inflammation and/or local tissue damage. Tendonitis, stress fractures, and ligament strains are just a few of the injuries caused by overuse.

Most pain you'll experience during exercise isn't life-threatening, but it can be serious. Painful ankles and knees might indicate muscle imbalance, not enough stretching, or worn-out shoes. Excessive and persistent fatigue or a feeling of continual heaviness may be your body's way of telling you that it is too stressed and that you need to slow down or take a few days off. In Chapter 23, "The Walking Wounded," I'll discuss specific injuries associated with walking, along with the care and prevention of each; but for now we will explore some of the more subtle warning signs for you to notice as you begin your walking career.

Overdoing Over-Training

Whoever thought that exercise could be unhealthy? Everything you read about, including the prevention and cure of disease and illness, mentions the many benefits of exercise and activity. Of course exercise is healthy … isn't it? The answer is yes and no. When you exercise excessively, you increase your risk of over-training. Over-training wears down your tissues and lowers your immune system, making you more susceptible to illness and injury.

Signs of over-training are sometimes very hard to detect because they often blend in with symptoms associated with other conditions not related to exercise. For example, one of the more common indicators that you might be over-training is insomnia. Yet the inability to fall asleep affects many, exercisers and non-exercisers alike. Other common symptoms are fatigue and depression. But again, these are common conditions among people who do not exercise, as well. Recurring injury, lack of appetite, or eating too much or too little are additional indications that you could be overdoing your exercise routine. Further in the chapter, I will discuss how to schedule regular breaks to prevent over training.

If the Shoe Fits ... or Not

In addition to sore feet, "bad shoes" can also cause problems with other parts of your body. When I say "bad shoes," I'm referring to shoes that don't fit properly, shoes that lack quality, or shoes that have been depleted of their cushion and absorbency. The problems they cause may start in the foot, but can travel up the leg to the knee, hip, and back, as well.

Discrepancies in footwear can knock off the balance of the rest of your skeletal system. Our body parts rely upon one another for stability and motion. We carry around a complicated system of biomechanical synchronicities underneath our skin and, whether you are aware of it or not, you are likely to shift your weight in an attempt to compensate for the disparity. This can cause muscle imbalances as well as uneven weight distribution and load in a particular joint or joints. In Part 5, "Your Feet," I discuss the injuries associated with improper footwear, as well as how to choose the right shoe.

Wise Walkers

Inspecting old shoes to see where the cushion of the sole wears down the most is like a map to your anatomy. It tells you where your limb and muscle discrepancies are. If you have pain on the inside or outside of your knee, for example, you might see excessive wear on the inside or outside of your sole. Similarly, the wrong-sized shoe may cause your foot to move around too much, or too little, disrupting the stability of the major joints in the body.

A Walk a Day Keeps the Doctor Away

Should you work out when you have a cold? How about if you have a fever? For many avid exercisers, especially beginners who have just managed to make walking a habit, stopping to give your body a rest can feel very threatening. You are afraid that if you stop, you may never start again. But there are certain circumstances when exercise can do more harm than good, especially when you are recovering from an illness like the common cold or the flu.

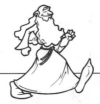

Wise Walkers

The common cold is just that: common. People suffer from colds twice annually, on average. Most doctors agree that moderate exercise is okay when fighting off a cold. Some may even promote it since it is believed to be beneficial to the healing process. Walking while getting over a cold is said to help speed up the recovery process because it gives the heart a jump-start, increases blood and oxygen flow through the body, and cleans extra mucus and other residue out of the lungs.

If you decide to exercise when you're stuffed up, make sure you really check with your body first. Do you feel excessive fatigue? How is your breathing? Does it feel difficult to fill your lungs as you normally would? Make sure you keep track of your pulse, both at rest and while you are working. If it seems unusually high, you might want to consider taking another day off.

If you do decide to take up the challenge, take it slower than usual. For example, even though it may be your day for hills, modify your schedule and keep it flat. If it's a "fast-pace" day, walk at a normal speed instead. Don't try to beat the clock this time. Finally, make sure you drink plenty of water. Hydration is crucial, especially when fighting off a cold. The following is a summary of guidelines you should follow if you decide to walk despite the sniffles:

➤ Wait until you are in the latter phase of your cold.

➤ Take your morning pulse; if it is 10 beats higher than normal, take another day off.

➤ Do a modified version of what you normally would do until you feel better.

➤ Start out slowly; if you feel okay, pick up the pace gradually.

➤ Drink plenty of water and make sure you get adequate rest.

➤ Listen to your body. If it doesn't feel right, then it probably isn't.

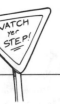

Walkers Watch Out!

Cortisol, the body's stress hormone, may suppress the body's immune function, thereby making you more susceptible to infectious diseases. That's why you are particularly vulnerable to colds and other illnesses when you're under pressure.

A simple stuffy nose is one thing, but exercising when you have a fever or other flu symptoms can be more damaging than good. Because a fever indicates that your body is fighting an infection, your immune system is on overdrive in an attempt to suppress the attacking virus. If you go out and exercise at such a time, you're putting even more strain on an immune system already under extreme stress as it attempts to fight off the intruder. Exercising will steal some of the energy away from the task at hand (healing) and could set your body up for a prolonged and more severe attack.

If it is the flu or a fever you suffer from, take time off! Wait until the illness has subsided. Be honest with yourself about how your body feels. Pushing yourself when you aren't ready will only drag the healing process out longer, setting your goal further and further back.

Unexplained Pain

Normal aches and pains associated with exercise are actually expected physical and psychological responses that occur when the body and mind are challenged. Minor aches and pains, *muscle soreness*, slight fatigue, thirst, a small increase or decrease of appetite, and moderate weight loss are just some of the symptoms you can expect a few weeks into your new exercise program.

On the other hand, pay attention to any unexplained and persistent pain unrelated to a previous injury, ill-fitting walking gear, or illness. Pain that has seemingly appeared out of nowhere and that has endured continuously for several weeks is a strong indication that you are dealing with a more serious problem than the "normal response to exercise" usually brings about. For example, bones that are unusually stiff might indicate that you have the beginning symptoms of arthritis or some other joint dysfunction. Roving muscle aches may be a warning sign of a muscle disease such as fibromyalgia. Unexplained weight loss or fever is often the first sign of the body's attempt to fight off some virus or bacterial infection.

Walkers Watch Out!

Be sure to take your temperature if you're unsure of your health status. When your body is under the weather and overtaxed, your heart rate will increase in an attempt to accommodate the suffering soma. If it has returned to normal levels (60 to 80 b.p.m.) then you have the green light to go ahead and exercise ... slowly!

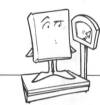

Weighty Words

Muscle soreness is also sometimes referred to as DOMS, Delayed Onset of Muscle Soreness. DOMS is thought to be a result of microscopic tearing of the muscle fibers. Swelling can occur in and around a muscle, which can also cause soreness hours later.

In addition to paying attention to the symptoms of injury or disease, you also want to be alert to more immediate signs that your body is in crisis.

Walkers Watch Out!

Any time you feel a sudden surge of dizziness, stop exercising and sit down. Wait for the feeling to subside. If it does not, have someone call 911. This could be the first signal of an oncoming heart attack. Shortness of breath and chest pain are other strong indications that you need to terminate activity and get in touch with an emergency health professional at once. Pain that shoots down the left arm is another important warning sign of a potential heart attack.

But I Don't Wanna!

It is inevitable that you'll experience days when you just don't want to exercise. You're too tired, too busy, too distracted, or just plain too uninterested to do anything strenuous today. That's pretty normal once in a while. However, if you dread your daily walk each and every time you step out the door, then maybe you'd better make some changes.

The truth is, it might just be time for a break. Most people would welcome a break, especially after a period of hard work. Rest is a time to relax, to rejuvenate, and to reward yourself for your efforts. But to many exercisers, especially those who have just managed to make it a habit, a "break" can be terrifying and more anxiety-ridden than relaxing.

To establish a habit, especially one that may not come naturally or that takes a lot of effort, we often must endure a period of intense discipline and self-control. Sometimes this rigid training is carried too far so that, even when we are well worthy of it, we don't dare take a break for fear that we might slip back into our previous habits and never be able to get off the couch again.

Unfortunately, not taking a break or giving yourself adequate rest could set you back in your goals despite your painstaking effort to avoid this. Whether you like it or not, you body needs rest. It needs time to rebuild, replenish, and refuel. It's imperative that you take a few days off whenever your body and—sometimes—your mind urges you to do so.

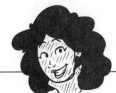

Interesting Excerpts

Feeling resentment, anger, anguish, or any other negative feelings about your walking program for a prolonged period of time is a good indication that you need a break.

No! Not Anytime You Feel Like It

On the other hand, just as over-exercising is a threat to the healthy progression of your walking routine, so is over-resting. Given the license to take a break, many people will carry it to the extreme and use it as an excuse not to follow their program. For this reason, it is important that you schedule breaks into your weekly workout. This way, you won't have to struggle with the decision of whether you should take the day off or not. The threat of turning one day of rest into 20 is extinguished, and you can relax with your weekly intermissions and maybe even learn to appreciate them a little.

So, exactly how much should you rest? The answer is quite simple—any time your body feels tired. But because "feeling tired" is such a subjective state of being, one that usually causes more confusion than clarity, I will give you a series of guidelines to follow:

➤ If you're a beginner, take a day off every other day. Try to limit your walks to three or four times per week.

➤ Intermediate walkers should try to take a day of rest every two days. Try not to walk "hard" two days in a row. For example, if you walk hills one day, try to walk flat the next.

➤ Advanced walkers can walk every day but, again, you should not push it each time. Try alternating between hard, medium, and easy days. Give yourself a rest once a week if possible.

➤ Listen to your body. If you feel fatigued and heavy, take the day off regardless of your schedule. If you continue to feel tired after two or three days of rest, then perhaps you are fighting off a virus and you need more time.

➤ Keep track of your morning pulse since it is the best gauge to determine the state of your body. Continually high morning heart rates may be telling you that your body needs a rest.

Wise Walkers

Yoga, or some other class that emphasizes flexibility, is a good substitute for "days off" if you don't feel comfortable with complete inactivity.

In the next chapter, we'll be going over sample programs for beginner, intermediate, and advanced walkers. I will explain ways to structure your weekly workouts so that break time is factored into the equation. The previous guidelines are just parameters to be aware of as you begin to design your own program.

Yes! You Can Do Other Activities; Substitutes in the Meantime

Taking a couple of days, or even a couple of weeks, off from walking doesn't mean that you have to succumb to a life of complete inactivity. Just because you may be a little burned out on walking doesn't mean you can't go for a swim or play a little tennis. Yes, it is important that you take a day or two off from exercise entirely each week, but you can also add other types of exercise into your schedule if you so desire.

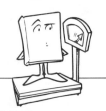

Weighty Words

Cross-training refers to incorporating more than one type of exercise into your weekly program.

Walkers Watch Out!

Don't give up if you take a break. Instead of looking at the break as something separate from your routine, think of it as something that is *a part* of it. Just before you start your walking routine again, reacquaint yourself with your goals if you feel your motivation meander. Remember, this is a part of your program, not a diversion from it.

In fact, *cross-training* can be considered a beneficial aspect of your walking workout for several reasons. For one, it adds variety to your exercise routine. Doing the same thing everyday can often become boring. By adding a day or two of some other form of exercise, you are not only breaking up your walking week but you also add a little spice to your program. You are also giving your muscles and your cardiovascular system a different type of challenge.

Taking an aerobics class, going for a swim, or doing yoga one or two times a week, in addition to walking, will help maintain balance in your body as well as in your exercise program. Not only will your muscles be challenged in a different way, so will your mind. Plus, you'll minimize the risk of developing an overuse injury—that is, an injury caused by using the same muscles and joints in the same movement over and over.

Motivating Yourself to Start Again

Starting up again after a long (or short) break can be a cause for concern for many. It doesn't have to be. Just because you've allowed yourself a little hiatus from your weekly walks does not mean that you have permanently slipped into your previous status of couch-us potato-us. The most important thing is that you plan ahead. Set a date. Circle a day on your calendar when you think you will be ready to start back again. Then let it go. Don't over-anticipate your return to walking. Try not to think about it too much. One of the problems with taking breaks is that people get overly anxious about their starting back up again.

They worry and fret so much over the possibility that they'll never be able to get back into the habit that they think themselves right into a rut.

Start to think of walking as something that you will be doing for as long as you can. When seen in this light, taking a break every once in a while doesn't seem so dramatic. After all, with an entire lifetime ahead of you, you'll have plenty of time to catch up, right?

The Least You Need to Know

➤ Persistent pain is a warning sign of injury.

➤ Walking with a cold is okay, but walking with the flu is not.

➤ It's okay to mix other exercise in with your walking program.

➤ A break every other day keeps the doctor away.

➤ Walking is a lifestyle, not a temporary fix.

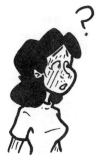
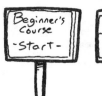

Chapter 10

In the Beginning

> ### In This Chapter
>
> ➤ Setting your goals
>
> ➤ Learning to plan ahead to avoid inevitable obstacles
>
> ➤ Rethinking your self-image
>
> ➤ How far, long, and hard?
>
> ➤ A sample program

It is one thing to understand the ins and outs of starting and maintaining a walking program; it is quite another to actually begin one. Up to this point, we have covered all of the major and minor details involved in setting up your walking routine—even in taking a break and watching out for injuries. By now, you are probably well-clothed and equipped with all the necessary accoutrements. You can recite the quantitative figures of your fitness-test results backward along with the pros and cons of every type of walking shoe available. Let's face it: You're ready!

In this chapter, we'll explore the specifics of designing a beginner's walking program. We will look at your past obstacles and ways to avoid them this time around. In addition to reiterating your goals, we will proceed step by step through a sample program that you may follow. Your time has arrived to move forward, so lace up your sneakers and let's get started!

New Kid Around the Block?

If exercise and, in this case, walking are entirely new to you, then chances are that you are feeling somewhat overwhelmed by now. You have learned a lot in the last nine chapters, and putting it into practice probably seems impossible at the moment. Not to worry. Learning new skills is always a challenge, but it promotes character and personal strength as well. So, go grab your goals and let's take a closer look at them before we start.

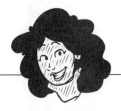

Goal Mining

Several chapters back, we discussed the advantage to establishing and following goals. Since then, we've discussed many things above and beyond the original reasons for beginning this fitness quest in the first place. Let's take a moment to reiterate your plans. As you know, goals are an important aspect of your fitness agenda because they help to keep you focused and directed. They serve as navigators through your fitness plight, helping to motivate and inspire you during the inevitable difficult and trying times we all experience at one point or another.

Once you've got your list of goals in front of you, ask yourself the following question: What exactly am I trying to achieve here? Many people summarize their desires in very general categories such as "lose weight," "tone up," or "get healthier." But what do these statements really mean to you?

Also, it is important that you be realistic. However hard you may try, if you were born with short legs, you cannot grow them longer by exercising. If you are genetically predisposed to large, short muscles, you probably will not develop a ballerina's body no matter how much you stretch. If your mother and her mother before her have wide hips, chances are that you will, too.

You must accept your body as it is and work with what you can. So, take a look at your goals one more time. Be honest with yourself and make modifications where appropriate. Following are some guidelines to help you pinpoint your long-term goals from your more general aspirations.

1. If your goal is to lose weight, how much? By what date? Generally speaking, you shouldn't expect to lose more than one or two pounds a week.

2. If you want to tone up, what part of your body are you trying to target? Would you like bigger shoulder muscles or less jiggle in your thighs? What date would you like to see this accomplished by?

3. If improving endurance is your aim, what type of endurance? Cardiovascular? Muscular? Would you like to be able to walk up Half Dome in Yosemite by late June, or take part in a marathon by May? Determine exactly what you mean by "improve endurance," and set a realistic date.

4. Perhaps improving your health is your aspiration. What indicates "improved health" to you? Lower blood pressure? If so, what measurement exactly? And by when? How about 30 points lower cholesterol in four months? Again, pinpoint your goals and attach a date to it.

Once you've managed to specify your long-term goals, you must break them down into smaller increments. Separate your goals into individual months, weeks, and even days. Stay in touch with the larger picture, your long-term goals, but focus daily on your smaller tasks. Getting caught up with the big changes may become overwhelming and too much to handle, causing frustration and non-compliance. Take it day by day and reward yourself often.

Wise Walkers

Substantial and permanent change takes time. You must be patient. Remember that these habits took a long time to establish and grow, so they are going to take some time to modify and change.

Be Proactive

Once you've established your goals, both long- and short-term, it is important that you are able to ease (rather than force) them into your lifestyle. Aspirations and ideals are good in theory, but putting them into practice is often the tough part. To avoid being overwhelmed by obstacles and lame excuses, it is best to be *proactive* and plan ahead. Start by taking a look at your calendar. Plan around events that might interfere with your goals. For example, if you normally walk on Mondays, Wednesdays, and Saturdays, but you've got an all-day conference coming up this Wednesday, plan your walk on Thursday or Friday instead. Know yourself and your habits. Be aware of those personal factors that have interfered with your progress in the past. Finally, take note of your psychology. Your mind is a very powerful tool that can work both for and against you.

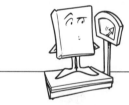

Weighty Words

To be **proactive** means to act in anticipation of future problems, needs, or changes.

Conscious Calendaring

Starting a new walking program is very exciting. You are finally doing something good for yourself and you should feel proud. But beginning a new program can also feel very precarious. Because this is something entirely new to you, and the habit has not yet been established, it is easy to get sidetracked and deterred from your original goal. Life and other "more important" responsibilities seem to always take over and interfere with your game plan. Before you know it, you are back to your old (walk-less) routine.

If you see that you have a major project coming up that has strict deadlines, make a commitment to yourself to get up a little earlier two mornings a week in order to take a brisk stroll around the neighborhood before getting ready for work. Or, have your assistant block off one hour, three days a week, in your schedule as an "appointment with self," and make sure the time is nonnegotiable. Without adequate preparation, your chances of drifting are greater. Remember that beginning any program, especially where exercise is involved, is going to be a little awkward and uncomfortable at first. Just be assured that with enough time and consistency, it will get easier.

Know Thyself

Working around your calendar is one thing; working around yourself is quite another. That is why it is very important to "know thyself" before setting up your program. For example, if you're the type of person who gets out of bed at 8 A.M. but does not actually wake up until noon, then chances are you are not a morning person. Setting your alarm for 6:30 A.M. for a morning walk will be like pulling teeth. If mornings are not your time, then schedule your walks for lunchtime, afternoon, or evening.

As you probably already know, change is difficult, so try to make changes one at a time rather than all at once. As you become more confident with yourself as a "walker," you can start to explore the possibility of changing your daily patterns around a bit; but for now, it is wise to just stick to the basics so you don't fail before you even begin. Here are some suggestions for working around some typical obstacles that might come up:

Walkers Watch Out!

Don't make it harder on yourself than it has to be. Because you are already challenging your patterns of physical activity, why add to the difficulty by changing your patterns of sleep and post-work relaxation as well?

➤ Not a morning person? Walk at lunch, after work, to and from work, or on the weekends.

➤ Have to pick the kids up after work? Take them to a park where they can walk (or play) with you before going home.

➤ Never get a chance to break for lunch? No time after work? Take a walk before your day starts to fill up. Get it out of the way first thing in the morning.

➤ You travel all the time in your job? Most hotels these days have gyms. If not, they certainly have stairs. Walk several flights of these instead.

➤ Don't have a full half-hour at a time to walk? Break it up into two 15-minute walks or three 10-minute walks.

These are just some of the many things you can do to work around your schedule. The point is that you have to want to make it work. Once you've decided this, then all obstacles become surmountable.

Psyching Out Your Psychology

Last, but not least, is the issue of your mind, your psyche—you know, the thing that Freud was all crazy about? Accepting yourself as a walker can be difficult, especially if you have not known yourself to be so in the past. We all have our preordained identities, and unfortunately these self-images tend to stick with us unless we work hard to challenge and change them. If you were overweight as a kid, for example, and not very active, it might be more difficult to see yourself as an athlete later on in life.

Perhaps you were the "girlie" type who viewed exercise as too masculine for your image. Maybe you always lived in the shadow of your more athletic and stronger older brother. Luckily, the beauty of human nature is that we can and do change. We have the ability to alter our thought patterns and to create new realities for ourselves if we work hard enough at it.

With this in mind, I think it's important to be extra aware of negative thought patterns as you begin your adventure into health. Make it a point to let go of fearful and doubtful thoughts that come up. It is probably impossible to erase all mental patterns immediately, but the more aware of them you are, the easier it will be to prepare for them. Replace negative thoughts with positive ones. Accentuate your small and larger accomplishments. Remind yourself of your achievements and stay positive as much as you can.

Avoid doubting Thomases. People who have nothing to offer but criticism and pessimistic input can be very poisonous and are likely to sabotage your plan if you are not careful. Seek people who offer inspiration and encouragement instead. Try not to over-analyze. The less you contemplate your motivation for change, the less likely you are to think yourself out of it. Just accept the new you and move on.

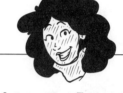

Interesting Excerpts

"Some of us are timid. We think we have something to lose so we don't try for that next hill."

—Maya Angelou (*USA Today*, March 5, 1988)

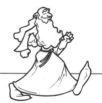

Wise Walkers

It is said that habits, both mental and physical, take three weeks to make and/or break. Give yourself at least this much time to change each pattern.

How Much? How Long? How Hard?

The most common mistake for novice (and experienced) exercisers is that they do too much too soon, and they end up injuring themselves or burning out before the month is over. As much as your enthusiasm is appreciated and needed, it must be appropriate if you want to establish a long-term habit. As I've mentioned earlier, it is best to start slow and to move forward conservatively. Adding days, time, and intensity is not as easy as 1-2-3; there is a system of progression that you should consider following if you want to stick with it (injury-free) for as long as you can.

How Much?

How often you exercise depends on your schedule and your level of fitness. But, generally speaking, it is a good idea to start out walking three days a week. If at all possible, try to skip a day (or two) between each workout since, particularly as a beginner, your body will need time to adjust to the new demands being asked of it. If you've managed to be consistent with your three days for a couple of months, add another day and again try to spread your workouts out. Try adding an extra day every four to six weeks or until your schedule does not permit. As I mentioned earlier, working out every day is okay, but it is always a good idea to take a day or two off. Ideally, you should set your program up so that you are walking three to five days a week with days off in between.

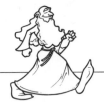

Wise Walkers

Just do it! Try to avoid getting too caught up in the details of time and scheduling in the beginning.

How Long?

Because walking is a relatively low-impact exercise, it may seem that you can walk forever. Chances are, however, that forever is not in your schedule, so try to limit it to no more than one hour. If you are completely new to exercise, you may even start out with 10 minutes and add a couple of minutes every week until you've reached 20 to 50 minutes. If time is an issue, you can always break yours down into segments. For example, if your goal is to walk 40 minutes four times a week, but you don't have that much time in one block, break it down into twice a day for 20 minutes each, or even three times for 15 minutes.

How Hard?

Perhaps the most significant factor to consider as a beginner walker is how hard you should walk. Americans have been raised to work hard and long, and we feel guilty if we don't. If you aren't suffering, then you aren't working hard enough, right? In some cases, this may be true; but when you are just beginning your walking program, you will definitely want to take it easy at first.

The emphasis in the beginning is not how hard you are walking but that you are walking at all. If you set up a program that has you feeling as though you are on the verge of exhaustion every time you finish, then chances are you will either drop out or get injured and have to quit. For this reason, I will not emphasize intensity for you beginners. For the first three months, try to keep your heart rate between 60 and 70 percent of your max. Don't walk so hard that you cannot carry on a conversation comfortably. Keep your routes flat and manageable.

The important factor, as a beginner, is to like what you are doing and to look forward to exercise rather than dreading it. If you're too hard on yourself in the beginning, you'll develop a negative association with exercise, and chances are you will eventually drop out. So, don't worry if you aren't sweating bullets or you aren't incredibly sore in the beginning. Your time will come for hard work, but not just yet.

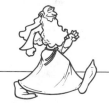

Wise Walkers

Just as a test, after a 10-minute warm-up, speed up your pace and try to walk as fast as you can. Maintaining this pace, now try to sing "The ABC's." Can't? This is what I mean by walking hard.

A Sample for an Example

Following is a sample six-month routine for you novice strollers. This does not mean that you must turn your schedule around completely to accommodate the following example. Instead, use it is a guide from which to gather ideas to design your own program or to follow until you get your own feet on the ground. The intensity portion of the chart refers to your heart rate. The numbers following are a percentage of your heart-rate max. Refer to Chapter 2, "One Step at a Time," for a review on percentages of your heart-rate maximum.

Sample Program for the Beginner

Weeks	Frequency	Duration	Intensity	Days
1 to 4	2 × week	10 min.	60%	M, Th
5 to 6	2 × week	15 min.	60 to 65%	M, Th
7 to 8	3 × week	15 min.	65%	M, W, Sat
9 to 10	3 × week	20 min.	65%	M, W, Sat
11 to 12	3 × week	20 min.	65 to 70%	M, W, Sat
13 to 14	3 × week	25 min.	65 to 70%	M, W, Sat
15 to 16	3 × week	25 min.	70%	M, W, Sat
17 to 18	4 × week	25 min.	65 to 70%	M, W, F, Sun

continues

Sample Program for the Beginner   (continued)

Weeks	Frequency	Duration	Intensity	Days
19 to 20	4 × week	30 min.	65 to 70%	M, W, F, Sun
21 to 22	4 × week	30 min.	70%	M, W, F, Sun
23 to 24	5 × week	30 min.	65 to 70%	M, T, Th, F, Sun

The preceding days are, again, just examples of how you might want to arrange the time. Your schedule may or may not be able to accommodate the one shown. Modify it as you see fit; just make sure you get out there and start moving!

Other Things to Keep in Mind

In case you haven't got enough to think about, here is one more thing to be aware of when beginning a walking program: You will feel sore. Chances are you will feel some minor aches and pains for the first several weeks. Do not be alarmed; this is just your body adjusting to the excess strain you are putting on it. Remember, you are breaking down your tissues and challenging a system that has become quite comfortable in its ways. It is only natural for your body to respond with a little discomfort at first. However, with time the pain will become less extreme as you become more used to the slight soreness one can expect when challenging their physical comforts.

One of the many benefits of exercise is increased overall energy. As your body becomes stronger, you will feel a general ease in the effort of everyday activities. But before you reach this point, expect an initial period of decline in your energy. Although this may not happen to everyone, fatigue is the body's natural response to a sudden rise in energy output. It takes time for it to catch up, and there may be a period when you find yourself feeling more tired than energetic. Don't let this discourage you. This will only last several weeks at the most. If you endure, you are sure to find a reciprocal reaction to occur, but you must be patient.

Walkers Watch Out!

Remember, pain and soreness are two different things. Anytime you feel any unexplained, sharp, and persistent pain, stop exercising and consult your doctor.

Change is uncomfortable at first, not only for you, but also for those around you. When starting anything new, try to be sensitive to the people you live with and how your change might be affecting them. Remember that walking takes time, sometimes away from someone else. If you and your spouse have spent the last 10 years watching your favorite sitcom together from 6 to 7 P.M. and you're now replacing the show with an evening walk, you might expect a little resistance and jealously from him or her. The best way to avoid this is to invite your spouse along. If he or she resists, then explain that this is not a move away from your time together but a step toward your health for your future together. With time, your spouse will get used to the change and may even decide to join you after all.

> ## The Least You Need to Know
>
> ➤ Specifying your goals is an important part of a successful program.
>
> ➤ Knowing yourself helps to avoid making unrealistic commitments.
>
> ➤ It's not how fast and how far, but rather, how to make walking a habit that counts.
>
> ➤ Soreness is a natural part of starting any physical regimen.
>
> ➤ Change can be hard for you and for others.

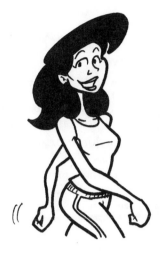

Chapter 11

And Now for the Rest of Ya!

In This Chapter

➤ How to know when you are ready to move forward

➤ Can you walk hills every day?

➤ Why intervals are back

➤ A sample program

➤ Why competing against others works

Perhaps the biggest question for any novice walker is how to know when you should take it to the next level. With so much emphasis on taking it slow and being conservative, it's no wonder you might be feeling a little apprehensive about moving forward. Your fears are understandable. Being impatient and jumping the gun with your fitness program can cause injury, fatigue, and burnout, and may ultimately sabotage your long- and short-term goals.

In addition to teaching you how to recognize when to take it to the next level, I will also show you ways to increase the intensity of your workouts. We will review the importance of hills and speed work, as well as the benefits of testing your skills against others. In this chapter, you will learn how to design your program so that you maintain balance and moderation while pushing the limits of your comfort zone. So, take a deep breath, and let's get going!

How to Know?

No two walkers are alike. Different people respond differently to the same type of exercise. Some of you, for example, may find that it has taken several months to increase your walking time from 15 minutes to 20 minutes without feeling tired. Others, on the other hand, were able to add five minutes to each walk every two weeks without any adverse effects. This doesn't mean that the latter are physically superior to the former. It simply means that their physiology is different. Age, body type, work schedule, prior fitness level, stress level, injury, and health history are all major factors affecting the rate of progression from one individual to the next.

For this reason, it's silly to think there's only one way for everybody to progress up the fitness ladder. If I'm not right there training beside you, how on earth can I know if you are ready to advance or not? This is a skill that you must learn to determine on your own. So, rather than my giving you orders on what to do, I'd rather focus on some of the physical changes that take place that tell you, the individual, when you are ready to take it to the next level.

Walkers Watch Out!

Did you know that when stress hormones are not turned off after stress, overexposure to these hormones wears on the body? That is why you may feel extra tired during your walks after an especially stressful work week.

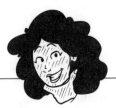

Interesting Excerpts

Knowing when to turn it up a notch is an important juncture for any beginner. It indicates that you've learned the skills to comprehend how your body works. Having a better understanding of your physical state is a difficult task to master, but by achieving it, you've brought yourself a lot closer to a healthier existence. Body awareness and moderation are key to maintaining a solid walking program because they help you recognize when you need to advance and when you need to cut back. Having this knowledge will help to promote a walking routine that is best suited to your body.

Let us start with your heart. Since you have been recording your *resting heart rate* for the past several months, you should be able to determine whether it has increased or decreased over time. As your heart gets stronger, it doesn't have to beat as often to deliver the same amount of blood throughout your body. If, after several months of sticking to your walking plan, you've noticed that your resting pulse is lower than it was when you first started out, then you know that your heart has gotten stronger and is ready for the next challenge.

Taking a closer look at the way you respond to exercise is a good way to determine your fitness level. If you feel like you can walk forever at 70 percent of your heart-rate max and still don't feel winded, then it is probably time for a program adjustment. If the four-mile walk to work no longer has you breaking out in a sweat, then chances are your cardiovascular system has improved. If you no longer feel a burn in your thighs by the second mile, this probably means that your muscle endurance has risen. The following is a summary of the signs and symptoms of a walker on the verge of transition:

➤ Lower morning pulse.

➤ Increase in overall energy.

➤ More stamina and ease of physical activities (walking up stairs, running for a bus, carrying groceries).

➤ Feeling like you can walk for longer at the end of most workouts.

➤ Little or no labored breathing with weekly walks.

➤ Needing concentrated effort to walk *slow* enough to maintain 60 to 70 percent of your HR max.

➤ Never feeling any discomfort.

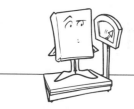

Weighty Words

Resting heart rate refers to a person's heart rate at rest. The best time to determine your resting heart rate is in the morning after a good night's sleep, just before you get out of bed.

If you feel like you've reached a plateau in the last several weeks and you no longer feel challenged by those walks that, at first, had you stopping for a breather every five minutes, then you know it's time to move into the world of the intermediate walker.

The Middle Man/Woman

You feel like a new person. You've been walking consistently three to five days a week for the past five to seven months, and you feel good. You would like to try something new and different but are unsure how to proceed? Chances are that you are ready to move to the next level and officially become an "intermediate" walker. Although no real terms or boundaries separate one type of walker from the next, you will pass through levels of fitness and experience as you advance in your pursuit as a walking wonder.

You can alter your program in several ways to meet the challenge your body is asking for. Picking up the pace and moving faster is the most obvious, of course, but certainly not the only way to increase your level of fitness. You can also add a day or two of hill walking to your weekly workout. Climbing an incline is not only harder for your lungs, but it works your legs in a different way as well. Another option is taking your walk to the track to do some interval training. Training at the track enables you to measure distance and time more objectively, and it can be very challenging (and fun), too.

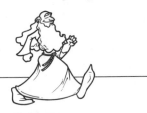

Wise Walkers

Now might be a good time to do your final fitness evaluation as a "beginner." Make sure that you keep all of your results together (and dated) so you can see how far you've come with each new phase.

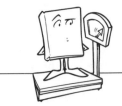

Weighty Words

Power walking is a term used to describe a fast walking pace—about 13 to 15 minutes a mile.

Pushing the Pace

The quickest way (literally) to add intensity to your walk is to pick up the pace. All you really need to do is to move your feet faster. That's it; nothing fancy. But exactly how much should you pick up the pace? And how will you be able to tell exactly how fast you are going? The simplest way to measure pace is by walking a clearly defined distance, such as a track. Walking around a track enables you to time your mileage down to the second. If you have a track available, I recommend starting there.

Start with a 10-minute warm-up at your normal warm-up pace. Once you're finished, walk the first lap at your regular pace. Time it. For the second lap, try to reduce the time by 30 seconds. Walk the third lap at your regular pace again, and the fourth at the faster speed. Alternate between the two until you've completed the time you've allotted for the workout (don't forget the cool down). To further increase the intensity, you can add another fast lap so that you're alternating between two fast laps with one regular one. Try adding a fast lap every other week until you're walking only fast laps.

If you do not have access to a track or a good stopwatch, you can use your regular route. If you're used to walking blocks, for example, time the first block, and then try to beat the next one by 30 seconds. Like the track workout above, alternate the blocks between the two paces. Substitute a regular block with a faster block each week until the entire walk is at the quicker pace. Stay here for a while before increasing your speed again; remember to spread out these harder walks since they can be intense workouts for your body (which will need a few extra days to recuperate).

If cutting your pace by 30 seconds isn't bringing your heart rate up enough, then pick up the pace even more and try to trim off a few more seconds. When you are measuring your heart rate, you will want to work somewhere between 75 to 85 percent of your heart-rate max. This doesn't mean that you'll need to walk at this pace for the entire walk—just the aerobic portion. After a 10-minute warm-up, start moving your feet faster until your heart rate has risen to 75 percent of its max. Stay here for a little while to see how your body adjusts to the intensity. If you still don't feel challenged, pick up the pace a bit to 80 percent and, again, stay there for a few minutes. Don't overdo it. Just because I've given you the license to advance doesn't mean that you should go all out. You still must be conservative with your progression. And you still must cool down after your workout.

Keep your terrain the same in the beginning. In other words, if you've been walking around your neighborhood, stick to your neighborhood. If you've been tracking it, then stay at the track. Shifting terrain, especially during higher-speed walks, could knock your balance (not to mention pace) off and cause you to twist an ankle. Try not to change too many things at once. Since you are already challenging your body to a new pace, adding a different terrain—and a whole new set of footwork—might only invite injury.

Finally, I strongly recommend balancing your weekly routine with both slower and faster days. If you are a three-times-a-week walker, substitute two of the days with faster days, while keeping the third one at a lower intensity. If you are walking four times a week, try walking faster two of those four days, leaving two days for a more relaxed stroll. Generally speaking, you should alternate between hard and easy days.

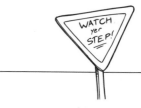

Walkers Watch Out!

Never compromise your safety for speed. Make sure you look both ways before crossing any street. Stop your watch in order to keep accurate time, but never try to zoom across a busy street just to stay "in time" with yourself.

Walkers Watch Out!

To avoid muscle soreness, you must start with easy to moderate activity and build up your intensity over time. Avoid making sudden major changes in the type of exercise you do and also in the amount of time that you exercise.

Making It Harder with Hills

Hills are another excellent way to raise the intensity of your walks. But hills, like speed, need to be implemented gradually into your weekly program. Suddenly adding a bunch of mountain climbs to your routine is likely to cause burn-out, fatigue, and injury. Try supplementing one day every three weeks. Choose a hill that is relatively low in grade and short in distance at first. Again, balance is the key here. Refer to

Walkers Watch Out!

Hill days and pace days are the same in that they both are "harder" workouts than usual. When designing your program, you should try to limit your harder days (hill or pace) to two to four (total) a week—no more. Mix up the two if you like.

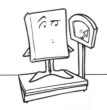

Weighty Words

Active rest refers to the lower-intensity intervals between each high-intensity interval. It is a time to rest your heart rate while you're still moving, rather than just stopping activity altogether (which can cause dizziness and fainting).

Chapter 6, "Now That You've Got the Basics, Let's Have Some Fun!" for some safety tips, as well as for form facts about walking hills, before you begin.

Implementing Intervals

Yet another way to add intensity to your walks is to interval train. Interval training is interspersed periods of high-intensity walking and lower-intensity *active rest*. When you interval train, you are pushing your pace anywhere between 15 seconds and several minutes. Although quite challenging, interval training can be very effective in advancing your level of fitness.

The best way to measure intensity during your interval training is by monitoring your heart rate. A heart-rate monitor is probably the most accurate means of doing this. By using one of these nifty little gadgets, you are more likely to get a closer reading of the number of heartbeats per minute than if you were to count your pulse. Refer to Chapter 2, "One Step at a Time," for a purchaser's guide on where and how much you should expect to pay for one of these "heart watches." If you decide not to purchase a heart-rate monitor, counting beats should be fine. Just make sure you are practiced at finding (and keeping) your heart rate to ensure an accurate count. Another important thing to have with you is a stopwatch, since you will be measuring your intervals by time. Try to buy one that has a digital readout, since these are often easier to see.

Interval training has three levels. The first one, sprint training, is the hardest as it requires you to work at the highest end of your maximum heart-rate capacity, usually somewhere between 90 to 95 percent. This level will increase your speed and power, but is impossible to maintain for long periods of time.

The second level is anaerobic threshold training, also known as *AT training*. During this phase, you will be working somewhere between 85 to 90 percent of your heart-rate max. At this level, you will increase your lactic-acid resistance in order for you to be able to walk faster and harder without stopping due to muscle fatigue. The anaerobic system is used most when walking up a hill at a relatively fast pace. You may find it difficult to speak at this level, and will definitely notice the burn in your thighs. Generally speaking, the harder you push yourself, the shorter your intervals will be.

In terms of the active rest portion of your intervals, generally speaking, the harder you push yourself, the more time you'll need for active rest. Correspondingly, the less

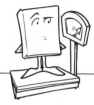

Weighty Words

AT training, also known as anaerobic threshold training, refers to working at an intensity high enough that oxygen can no longer supply the need for energy. Ever heard of the term "run out of breath"? Well, this is literally what happens when the need for oxygen from the working muscles exceeds the speed at which the heart can deliver blood to them. The muscles need something to fuel them so they turn to stored energy, in the form of sugar, to keep them going. This is the anaerobic system.

you push, the shorter your active rest periods should be. For sprints and anaerobic intervals, you'll want to give yourself anywhere from two to five minutes. For aerobic intervals, you need only between 30 seconds to two minutes. The following is a summary of the different levels of interval training as well as the heart-rate percentages and times that correspond with each.

Interval	HR%	Time/per	Active Rest
Sprint	90 to 95%	10 to 30 sec.	3 to 5 min.
Anaerobic	85 to 90%	30 to 90 sec.	2 to 5 min.
Aerobic	75 to 85%	2 to 5 min.	30 sec. to 2 min.

Also, you will want to start with only a few intervals at a time. I recommend doing no more than three to five intervals per workout when you first begin. Any more might be too hard on your body and cause injury. Try adding one interval every two weeks. You don't really need to do more than 10 intervals per workout, particularly if you are sprinting. You can also mix up the types of intervals if you'd like, so that a third of them are sprints, a third are anaerobic, and a third are aerobic.

Finally, because you are pushing your body harder than usual, it is crucial that you spend an ample amount of time stretching after you do interval training. Your muscles will be extra tight from all the power-work and will need added care as a result.

A Sample Week

Now that you have all this information, how on earth are you supposed to put it all together into an organized and coherent fashion? You like the idea of climbing hills to work your buns a little more, but the interval training sounds fun, too. You've wanted to increase your pace for a while now, but you're not sure how to fit it all in. Designing and planning your walking routine can seem complicated at first, which is why I have designed the following sample week. Whether you are a three-day-a-week walker or an everyday stroller, having the correct balance between hard and easy days is crucial for progressing effectively and safely without injury.

Sample Weekly Workouts

Total Walking	Monday	Tuesday	Wednesday	Thursday	Friday	Saturday	Sunday
3 days	pace	*off*	easy	*off*	hill	*off*	*off*
4 days	pace	*off*	hill	easy	*off*	int	*off*
5 days	*off*	int	easy	hill	*off*	pace	hill
6 days	pace	easy	hill	*off*	int	hill	easy
7 days	pace	easy	hill	easy	int	easy	hill

The preceding table is all-inclusive. If, however, your goal is to just increase your speed, you can substitute the hill days with pace and interval days. If you want to climb Mount Shasta in six months and you want to strengthen your hiking legs, feel free to replace the pace days with hill days. The important thing is to balance your hard workouts with easy ones. It would be a good idea to spend a little extra time stretching after each hard workout as well. Finally, listen to your body and take a break if you're feeling depleted and tired (despite the fact that it's not a "rest day" on your pre-programmed schedule).

Comparing with Competition

If you feel like you have reached your endurance and pace goals and cannot increase your speed anymore, but would like to find out how you compare to others in your age group, then perhaps you are ready for your first competition. Just like runners, walkers have events that put their fitness to the test, be it speed, time, or distance. This is a good time to home in on your goals and to become a little more disciplined with your routine. Working toward a goal in which you compete against others can be a very inspiring and motivating event. Although competition is not limited to the "advanced" walker, it is a good way for you, as an intermediate walker, to test all your hard work and take your fitness to the next level.

Goal-Setting for the Advanced Walker

At this stage in your walking career, specific goal-setting is an important component in your success. At first you might have focused on general fitness, health, and weight loss, but now all your hard work and diligence can be put to the test in one specific event. Deciding to compete is a big and exciting step. It is important to choose an event that is within your limits. However proud you may be of your dedication and progress, competing in an event that you are not ready for can be detrimental to your success as a competitor (and as a walker).

The best course of action to take at this point is to look through your local sports magazine or newspaper. Underline and write down the events that interest you. Mark them on your calendar and take the time to check them out as a viewer rather than as a participator. Get a feel for the lay of the land, the cast of characters, and the general ambiance. Ask yourself if this is something you want to take on. Visit several races and events to get an idea of how they differ from one to the next.

If you are still intrigued by the idea of competing and would like to give it a try, look ahead at your calendar and find a time that is not too crazy in terms of work and social events. Planning your first competition during the holidays, for example, is not a good idea. Also, be realistic. Don't set your sights on a marathon the first time around. Training for such events can be very time-consuming and hard on your body; if your introduction into competition is an extra painful one, then chances are that you will not want to continue. Please refer to Chapter 20, "Taking It to the Next Level," for a more detailed discussion of your transition into the world of competitive walking.

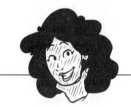

Interesting Excerpts

While Russians claim the most Olympic walking medals to date, Larry Young from the United States has won more Olympic medals than any other American walker.

Wise Walkers

One does not have to actually compete in a walking event. If you do not feel like racing against time, you may enter an event that allows all levels of walkers to participate, so you can take part without the pressure of time at your back.

The Least You Need to Know

➤ Change is difficult and uncomfortable at first.

➤ Hills and speed-work are two sure ways to increase your fitness level.

➤ There are no clear-cut differences between intermediate and advanced walkers.

➤ Adding competition to your program is a good excuse for discipline.

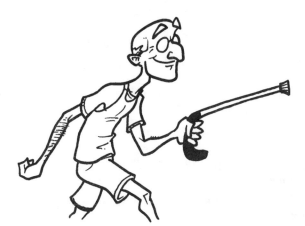

Chapter 12

Walking for Special Populations

In This Chapter

➤ How to fight the aging process

➤ Why inactivity can make arthritis worse

➤ Dealing with diabetes through movement

➤ Why physical inactivity is a major risk factor for heart disease

➤ Modifying exercise programs to fit your lifestyle

Exercise is not only for those looking to stay healthy; exercise also works for those who are trying to *become* healthy. In fact, it serves as one of the most inexpensive and effective "medications" for many health conditions, including diabetes, high blood pressure, heart disease, and arthritis. Plus, it helps to keep you feeling young and vital, too!

It is never too late to start a walking program. People of all ages and with most types of ailments can benefit from exercise. Beyond the fact that it does indeed improve your health, it also livens up your spirit. Walking gives you a sense of dignity and pride as you take constructive steps to improve your welfare. In this chapter, we'll explore several health conditions that you can improve with just a little bit of walking each week. We'll also look at ways to modify your program to fit your needs, as well as highlight precautions you should take to ensure a healthy, happy journey.

The Silver Saunter: How Walking Helps with Aging

Unfortunately, growing older in our society is seen by some as a handicap. But it doesn't have to be that way. Staying physically active and keeping your body in motion is one of the best ways to ease the aging process. Balance and agility are skills that are learned and that diminish without practice, regardless of your age. Poor balance, weak bones, loss of agility—you can avoid all of these "old people" characteristics with just a little activity every day.

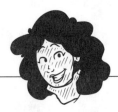

Interesting Excerpts

Thirty-one million people, or 12 percent of the total U.S. population, are aged 65 and older. The Census Bureau anticipates that 62 million people will be aged 65 and older by 2025.

Wise Walkers

Physical exercise can reverse about half of the physical decline normally associated with aging. In fact, many of the symptoms associated with "aging" actually have little to do with growing old per se, but rather are linked to lack of muscle use that leads to muscle atrophy.

Although certain physical changes are bound to occur as a result of aging, they don't have to be debilitating. In the following section, we will review some of the more common negative associations with growing older and how developing an active lifestyle helps us overcome them.

Osteoporosis: Battling Brittle Bones

Osteoporosis is a decrease in the density of bone mass. As we age, our bones become weaker and more brittle due to, among other things, the decline of physical activity that tends to come with aging. Our bones need load and pressure on them in order to stimulate growth. With a decrease in weight-bearing activity, they lose their strength and become more susceptible to fractures. Because the risk of bone injuries rises with age, older people become more timid and even less mobile for fear of hurting themselves. Of course, this only perpetuates the problem since it is the bearing of weight that our bones need in order to keep them strong.

Poor diets and lack of appropriate nutrition add to the decline of our bones' strength as well. Loss of appetite and interest in food robs our elders of important vitamins and minerals such as calcium and vitamin D, whose functions are to keep our bones strong and healthy. When you're not eating right, your energy declines, leaving you tired and listless and completely unmotivated to move, which, needless to say, perpetuates the problem even further.

Adding bouts of light activity and weight training several days a week can make a world of difference to the formation of bone mass. Weight training and other physical activity causes the muscles to pull on the bones, which stimulates growth. The more weight-bearing activity you put on your body, the greater the production of bone strength. And the more actual load you place on the skeletal system, the stronger the bones become. At the end of this chapter, I will provide a progressive workout geared toward an older population, with modifications for each special age-related condition. But for now, start thinking about ways that you might modify your lifestyle to prevent osteoporosis. The following are some suggestions to consider:

1. Increase the activity in your everyday life within and around the home (walking stairs, gardening, walking to grocery store).

2. Review your diet to see where you might implement more calcium- and vitamin D-rich foods.

3. Do not skip meals.

4. If you are a woman approaching menopause, ask your doctor about estrogen therapy.

5. If you smoke, stop.

6. Decrease your consumption of alcohol.

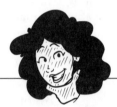

Interesting Excerpts

Another bone-related problem that results from a lack of activity is stiffness caused by poor joint nutrition. Physical activity helps to bring fluid in and out of your joints. Movement helps bring nutrients into the bone structure and to move waste products out. This keeps the joint structure properly lubricated, allowing your bones to stay healthy and strong. If you do not move enough, however, your joints will not receive the nutrients they need to function properly. The connective tissue around them becomes stiff and brittle, which only serves to limit the movement of the joint even more.

Practicing Proprioception

Another common problem among older adults is a decline in proprioceptive consciousness. Proprioception simply means the awareness of our bodies (and its movement) through space. Unfortunately, balance is a major concern for many older adults. Broken hips are often due to a fall caused by a loss of balance. Muscle strength

131

and endurance, along with the compliance of connective tissue, decline rapidly with age, causing many older adults to feel less agile and in control of their bodies. As a result, they do not feel as secure on their feet. Unfortunately, the less you use the skills, the less comfortable you feel with them so that, eventually, you become almost entirely sedentary, perpetuating the problem even further.

By walking, you're practicing the skill of proprioception. Walking does not appear to be an activity that requires a lot of coordination, but in fact it does. Moving one foot in front of the other while being able to judge depth and space takes skill and control. Whether you are aware of it or not, being able to walk while looking ahead, not down, means that you are relying on your peripheral vision to keep you alert. Obviously, the more you walk, the better you become at judging depth and space, and the more comfortable you feel on your feet.

Maneuvering Your Muscles

If you feel less stable on your feet, chances are you'll move less. In addition to losing important bone mass, you risk losing muscle strength and endurance as well. Ever heard of the saying, "use it or lose it"? That's what will happen with your muscles as you sit there motionless all day long. Muscle *atrophy* is the inevitable result of a sedentary lifestyle. Why should a muscle maintain its vigor if it's not being used? The following is a list of things that happen when your muscles are inactive:

➤ Loss of muscle endurance, making everyday activities more tiresome

➤ Loss of muscle strength, which puts more pressure on your joints

➤ Loss of muscle elasticity and flexibility, which causes muscle tightness, thereby increasing your risk of injury

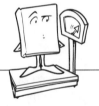

Weighty Words

Atrophy comes from the Greek word *atrophos*, which means "ill fed." It is the decrease in size or wasting away of a body part or tissue.

Walking helps to build and maintain overall muscle efficiency. It tones and increases muscle strength and endurance while keeping them pliable and supple. As you move more, your body responds by building more muscle tissue. With more muscle comes an increase of oxygen and nutrition flowing through your system, which helps to maintain its productivity and stamina. Daily activities become easier and more manageable, which promotes a sense of well-being and liveliness. A higher sense of self-confidence enables you to feel more independent and competent. You see, our bodies are very adaptable organisms no matter what our age, and if treated properly they will respond accordingly.

Getting Your Doctor's Approval

Now that I've convinced you that starting a walking routine can make your life easier, more enjoyable, and healthier, you must do a couple things before rushing out to pound the pavement. First and foremost, you must get your doctor's approval. Even though you may not have any known medical condition, it is still imperative that you go in for a physical and get an A-OK from Dr. Feel Good. In fact, the American College of Sports Medicine strongly recommends that all men over the age of 45 and all women over the age of 55 should see their doctor before starting any exercise routine. So, make sure you make an appointment before you do anything else. Besides, it's a good way to collect all the physical data you'll need to start your notebook.

What Is Arthritis and How Does Walking Help?

Arthritis literally means "joint inflammation," and it affects one out of seven people, according to the Arthritis Foundation. More than half of those people afflicted with arthritis are over the age of 65, but it does occur in younger people as well. Extreme stiffness and swelling of the joints causes immense pain, which results in inactivity and joint damage. As you can see, a vicious cycle ensues, leaving you feeling even more helpless against the problem.

Because inactivity seems to be the only way to avoid the pain, muscles and connective tissues become weaker from lack of use. Joint degeneration increases as you place more pressure and load on them rather than on the muscles. Simple everyday activities like lifting yourself out of bed, getting dressed, or climbing in and out of the car become arduous and unmanageable.

Painful Beginnings

Sounds bleak, doesn't it? Well, it doesn't have to be. Once believed to be the culprit of arthritic problems, exercise is now believed to be the saving grace for those with painful joints. Regular movement is said to decrease the swelling of the joints

Wise Walkers

Only 8 percent of the adults in the United States currently exercise at recommended levels. The Center for Disease Control and Prevention estimates that 92 percent of American retirees do no meaningful exercise and that one half of American retirees are sedentary.

Wise Walkers

Did you know that there are over 100 types of arthritis? Such conditions include, but are not limited to: rheumatoid arthritis, osteoarthritis, Reiter's Syndrome, gout, juvenile arthritis, and Lyme Disease.

and to minimize the pain that occurs with arthritis. Exercise also helps to rebuild muscle strength and connective tissue, thereby lifting some of the pressure (and pain) off the bones. Being physically active promotes weight loss so you carry less weight on your joints as well. Finally, movement promotes nourishment and waste-product removal to and from the joint, keeping it healthier and more pliable.

If you are suffering from arthritis, you must remember that starting out is going to be uncomfortable. Because you probably have not moved your body much, it will feel stiff and unyielding in the beginning. This is why walking is such an ideal way to introduce yourself to activity. In fact, due to its low-impact nature, walking serves as one of the best forms of exercise for the arthritic. As the blood and oxygen flow through your body, you will notice a general ease in the way you move as your joints and bones become healthier and stronger.

Begin with just a few minutes at a time. Find a flat surface and start out slowly. Forget about pace, time, calories, and the like. Just allow your body to move naturally. If you need to sit down to take a break, go ahead. If you feel too much pain, stop and try again the next day. If walking on concrete feels too painful, try walking on a softer surface, or walk in a swimming pool. Water will alleviate some of the body weight and pressure from your joints, making it less painful.

Walkers Watch Out!

If the joint feels hot, it most likely means that it is inflamed. Do not exercise with joint irritation. Wait until the inflammation has subsided before exercising.

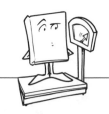

Weighty Words

Hyperglycemia is a condition that is often associated with diabetes, a condition in which too much glucose is in the bloodstream due to a lack or inefficiency of the hormone insulin. Signs of hyperglycemia are a great thirst, a dry mouth, and a need to urinate often.

Diabetic and Dynamite

Diabetes is a disease that prevents the body from processing sugar properly due to insufficient insulin function. Insulin acts as a vehicle for carrying sugar (glucose) into, as well as out of, the body. When you don't have enough glucose—fuel—being transported through the bloodstream, the cells do not receive the adequate nutrition they need to function properly. On the other hand, when you have too much glucose in the bloodstream, you're at risk for a condition known as *hyperglycemia,* which can have an adverse affect on your blood vessels, nervous system, and other tissues.

Unfortunately, diabetes is on the rise in the United States, with more than 10 million adults and more and more children suffering from the disease. Why are so many Americans diabetic? One of the main reasons is poor diet and lack of exercise. With the increase of high-fat and sugary foods, not to mention immense portion sizes and an increasingly sedentary lifestyle, it is no wonder that so many of us are at risk for the disease. As we become more obese and less healthy, our bodies become less sensitive to the influence of insulin.

Walking Your Sugar Down

Fortunately, something can be done about controlling diabetes. Studies have proven that with the addition of regular exercise and a balanced diet, you can bring your diabetes under control and expect to live a long and healthy life. Walking helps in several ways. First, it controls blood glucose levels by enabling the body to take glucose out of the bloodstream and to use it as fuel for exercise. Second, it increases your body's sensitivity to the use of insulin. Third, muscle contraction stimulates the transport and absorption of glucose into the bloodstream. Finally, it decreases body fat and obesity, which improves insulin sensitivity and promotes homeostasis. The following is a list of guidelines to follow as you start your quest for better health:

1. Use proper footwear and, if appropriate, other protective equipment.
2. Inspect your feet daily and after exercise (those with diabetes may have wounds that heal more slowly than they would for others).
3. Check insulin levels before, during, and after exercise if possible.
4. Avoid exercise during periods of poor metabolic control.
5. Carry insulin with you.
6. Carry an ID bracelet on you that describes your diabetic condition.
7. Avoid exercise in extreme heat or cold.
8. Exercise with a partner if possible.
9. Have a high-carb snack handy.

At the end of this chapter, I will go into more detail about duration, frequency, and intensity for the diabetic walker.

Diet Do's and Don'ts

Although exercise is very effective in controlling the disease, you must also be aware of the food choices you make as well. After all, it is bad eating habits that got you here in the first place, right? Visit your local Center for Diabetes if there is one available. Many of these centers offer seminars and classes on ways to change your diet and your lifestyle to adapt healthier habits. Talk to your doctor as well; he or she may be able to recommend a national organization, such as the American Diabetes Association, to give you more information (see Appendix A, "Resources for Walking Fit").

Walking for the Cardiac Rehab Patient

Heart disease is the leading cause of death in America. Each year more than 500,000 people die from heart attacks due to coronary artery disease. Also known as CAD, coronary artery disease is the culprit of several heart-related conditions such as angina, heart attack, and congestive heart failure. Just as many women die of heart disease as men, especially after menopause when levels of the heart-protecting hormone estrogen, drop significantly. Poor diets and obesity, inactivity, high stress, and cigarette smoking are the other leading causes of heart failure.

The coronary arteries carry blood to the heart. Blood serves as food and energy so that the heart can function properly. Insufficient blood supply is due to clogged arteries. Arteries are clogged by something known as *plaque*. An abundance of plaque build-up over time hardens and restricts blood flow through the artery walls. When an insufficient amount of blood (fuel) is being delivered to it, the heart has to work harder. Eventually the heart weakens and performs less efficiently. Breathlessness, irregular heart rhythms, excessive fatigue, and heart attack are all symptoms of a weakened heart.

Walkers Watch Out!

According to the American Heart Association, more than 1,100,000 Americans will have a new or recurrent coronary attack, and more than 40 percent of the people experiencing these attacks will die of them this year.

Heart disease is something that creeps up on you. Poor lifestyle choices and a genetic predisposition slowly destroy your blood vessels without notice. You may carry on in a relatively normal manner until suddenly you experience severe chest pain and heart failure. Fortunately, many of the culprits that cause coronary artery disease are environmental and can therefore be controlled. The following is a list of some of the risk factors associated with heart disease:

1. Age: men over 45 years, and women over 55 years

2. Heredity: male family member diagnosed with heart disease before the age of 55, and female family member diagnosed before the age of 65

3. Gender: men at mid-life, and women after menopause

4. Physical inactivity

5. Cigarette smoking

6. High blood pressure

7. High cholesterol

8. Stress

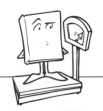

Weighty Words

Plaque is the deposit of fatty substances, cholesterol, cellular waste products, calcium, and other substances in the inner lining of an artery.

9. Diabetes

10. Obesity

The preceding risk factors mentioned are primarily ones that can be altered given some time. Becoming physically active is perhaps one of the most important ways to begin, since inactivity is one of the leading causes for many of the other risk factors listed. Whether you are struggling with some form of heart disease or just would like to take the necessary precautions to avoid it, exercise should be a regular part of your program back to health.

How Walking Helps

Exercise is one of the most useful tools in improving your overall health. Walking keeps your muscles and connective tissue supple and healthy while giving your heart the necessary challenge to make and keep it strong. It keeps your blood vessels pliable and strong, allowing more blood to flow through them. It can increase the amount of capillaries, which increases the exchange of nutrients, oxygen, and waste products to and from the muscles. It increases your levels of good cholesterol (HDL) while lowering the levels of bad cholesterol (LDL), which is a major component of plaque build-up in the arterial walls. In addition, it enhances your body's sensitivity to insulin levels, thereby decreasing your risk of diabetes, another major risk factor for CAD. Finally, it helps to promote healthier behavior such as smoking cessation and weight loss, two other conditions that are high on the list as risks for heart disease.

Heart-Rate Monitors and Supportive Supervision

If you've suffered a heart attack or have been diagnosed with a heart condition such as ischemic heart disease or angina, then you must first complete the cardiac rehabilitation portion of your recovery before beginning an exercise program on your own. Classes and other educational programs are usually offered by the health facilities where you were initially treated. Medical supervision is a must during the first several weeks and months of your recovery, especially because the heart is in a precarious state and needs to be monitored closely.

Once you have been let loose into the world, taking with you all of the information you learned during your rehabilitation, you might want to start by doing several things. First, I suggest purchasing a heart-rate monitor. This way you will be able to keep close tabs on your heart rate as you go. Second, enlist the company of a walking partner. Although you may be feeling strong and healthy, it is always a good idea to have supervision during the first several weeks and months of beginning your exercise program in the unlikely event that something goes wrong. Third, enroll in a continuing-education class that offers support and education for those who have suffered a heart attack or have been diagnosed with heart disease. This will not only serve as a way to keep you updated on all the latest studies, but also can be used as a tool to

Walkers Watch Out!

Please note that certain heart medications can alter your heart rate. If you are taking such a medication, use the talk test to determine the intensity of your effort instead.

prevent noncompliance. The American Heart Association is an invaluable resource. I suggest you take the time to research their online site at www.american-heart.org.

First and foremost, you must start out slow. Due to the susceptible state of your heart, you must take care in adding only bits of activity at a time. Try walking just five minutes every other day to get used to the feel of the exercise. Once you feel comfortable with this, add a day or two so that you are walking 5 to 7 days a week for 5 to 10 minutes. Work up to 20 to 30 minutes 5 to 7 days a week by adding 5 minutes every other week. This may seem excruciatingly slow, but it is always better to be safe than sorry. Also, stay close to home base at first, or at least a populated area, so that help can be contacted if necessary.

Warning Signs While Walking

For the most part, walking is probably one of the best forms of exercise you can choose, for several reasons. First, it's easy. Because you've been doing it for the better part of your life, walking takes very little skill and coordination. Second, it's efficient. No expensive equipment is needed, except a decent (and comfortable) pair of walking shoes. Finally, it's easy to monitor. If you feel too overworked, you can slow down and take a breather. Plus, it's continuous and flowing, which helps to establish regular breathing patterns—an important factor for the recovery of your heart's health.

There is, however, a slight chance that walking, on any form of exercise for that matter, might exacerbate your heart condition as well. Below is a list of warning signs that you should be aware of:

➤ Abnormal heart rhythm

➤ Chest pain, pressure, or tightness

➤ Shortness of breath or difficulty in breathing

➤ Dizziness, lightheadedness, or cold sweats

➤ Excessive fatigue

➤ Pain down the left arm

If you experience any of these symptoms during your jaunt, stop and call 911 immediately! There is a chance you might be suffering another attack, so getting to the emergency room as quickly as possible is imperative.

The Least You Need to Know

➤ Walking and exercise improve functional abilities in older adults.

➤ People with arthritis benefit from moving their bodies daily.

➤ Walking helps those with diabetes control their blood sugar.

➤ An inadequate supply of blood to the heart weakens it and eventually can result in a heart attack.

➤ Increasing your activity level eliminates 7 out of the 10 risk factors associated with heart disease.

Part 3

Walking for Weight Loss

If weight loss is your primary motive for starting a walking program, then you've come to the right place. Walking is one of the easiest exercises for dropping pounds and inches because it's so simple to do. Walking is also great for those carrying around extra pounds because it's a low-impact sport, and therefore is easy on the joints. In this part, I'll show you ways to get out of the rut of past failures by changing your attitude about exercise. You'll discover ways to set realistic goals, why diets don't work, how to increase the intensity of your walks, and suggestions for changing bad habits into good ones.

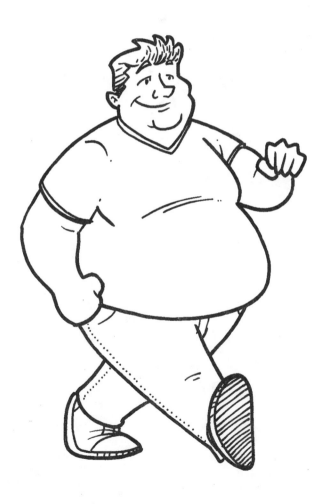

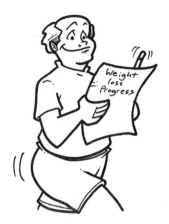

Chapter 13

Weight Walkers

In This Chapter

➤ Obesity as a major health problem in the United States

➤ How to overcome psychological barriers

➤ Redefining your goals

➤ Suggestions for overcoming old obstacles

➤ Making motivation work for you

Starting a weight-loss program isn't necessarily a very difficult task to take on. Sticking to a weight-loss regimen, however, is an entirely different matter. And keeping the weight off once it's been lost is nearly impossible for most. Despite our apparent obsession with thinness, weight loss, and diets, America is growing fatter by the year. In fact, annually, more than 30 billion dollars are spent on weight-loss pills and diet paraphernalia. According to the American Obesity Association, over 55 percent (97 million) of Americans are considered obese today. Obesity is the second-leading cause of unnecessary deaths and is an independent risk factor or an aggravating agent for more than 30 medical conditions.

Maintaining a healthy weight is indeed essential. However, before you start beating yourself up over your extra girth, keep in mind that it isn't all your fault. Today's society is a fast-paced one that encourages you to eat more junk food on the go—and when you can finally relax, you naturally want to take it easy in front of the television rather than exert more energy to exercise. But in this chapter, I'll help you meet your goal of losing weight while showing you that adding a walking routine into your life will give you more, not less, energy.

Weight-Related Diseases and How Walking Helps

We are a large nation filled with large people. In fact, at least 97 million Americans have been diagnosed as being *obese*. Obesity is responsible for 300,000 deaths in the United States each year, costing the country more than $100 billion annually. Being overweight can cause a whole host of problems, both physical and psychological.

Heart disease, high blood pressure, high cholesterol, depression, diabetes, structural problems, and general discomfort are just some of the adverse conditions associated with obesity.

As I mentioned earlier, walking helps to reduce most, if not all, of the symptoms mentioned above. First and foremost, walking increases your energy output. Increased energy output equals more caloric expenditure, which leads to weight loss. As you feel better, chances are you will begin to modify your diet and eat better. Cutting out fatty foods, high sugar, alcohol, and salt will minimize your risk for diseases such as diabetes, CAD, high blood pressure, and high cholesterol. As you begin to treat yourself better, you will feel more confident and in control of your life. Where once you may have shied away from social events, now you will embrace them. Depression and anxiety that formerly dominated your moods will slowly start to subside and you will begin to feel normal again.

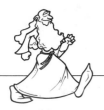

Wise Walkers

Remember that body fat and body weight are two different things. Two people may weigh the same on the scale, but the one with lower body-fat percentage is not only going to appear thinner but will also be healthier.

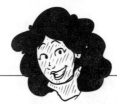

Interesting Excerpts

Scientists have discovered that there are certain chemicals in the brain called neurotransmitters that influence what we eat. The amount of these chemicals in our blood or brain fluids corresponds to certain cravings we experience. If we lack a certain type of protein consumption neurotransmitter, for example, we might crave meats and dairy products. Neurotransmitters also control our eating behavior in that they influence when we start eating, how long we eat, how fast we eat, when we stop eating, and how long the interval between eating will last.

Psychological Barriers and Social Shyness

I am not implying that starting a weight-loss and exercise regimen is as easy as 1-2-3. Chances are you've stopped and started many diets and exercise attempts over the years, none of which ever seemed to work. It is no wonder that with so many failed efforts, you would feel apprehensive and hesitant about any words of advice I might have to offer. And I don't blame you. Making changes can be very intimidating and awfully frustrating, especially if you don't succeed the first several times.

If you're like most of the beginning exercisers and dieters today, the chances are that you will quit within several weeks after beginning your program if you don't see results immediately. But the body (and mind) takes time to change. There are no pills, potions, or quick fixes when it comes to health and fitness. You must work at it, and work at it consistently, and then wait patiently for the results. And they will come *if* you give them time to.

First you must overcome the psychological barriers preventing you from starting and sticking to an exercise program. Then you must challenge the social issues that come up if you are overweight and uncomfortable with your body. Many heavy people feel self-conscious about exercising in public. You may feel like you are being watched and even ridiculed by your more fit peers. If you feel extremely self-conscious and shy about exercising in public, then it's going to be virtually impossible to keep your commitment to yourself.

You must realize that everyone had to start somewhere. No one was "born" to run, but had to work at it and build this skill over time. Starting is perhaps the most difficult aspect of taking on anything new, as you are learning skills and a whole different way of thinking that do not come naturally to you. And your challenge is even greater as you struggle with the stigma attached to being overweight. However real it may seem, the chances are that people are not being as judgmental as you fear. Enlist the help of a friend if this will ease your discomfort when first starting out. Join a support group of

Wise Walkers

According to the American Heart Association, the incorporation of exercise into a person's permanent lifestyle increases the likelihood of long-term success in weight loss. Regular exercise also helps to increase energy expenditure, maintain lean body mass, improve functional capacity, reduce cardiovascular risk, and promote a sense of general well-being.

Walkers Watch Out!

If the idea of getting on the scale, measuring your limbs, or determining your body-fat percentage fills you with dread and fear, skip them. This is the beginning of a positive change, not one that is supposed to make you feel apprehensive.

people who are struggling with the same issues. Remember that starting anything new is going to be awkward and disconcerting at first, but these feelings will subside the longer you stick to it.

Setting Your Short- and Long-Term Goals

Establishing long- and short-term goals to "get fit" is one thing, but determining goals for weight loss is yet another. Because weight loss is such a difficult task for most, it is imperative that you spend some time focusing on exactly how and what you would like to achieve. Simply "losing weight" will not be a strong enough objective to keep you motivated. Skipping meals, cutting out sweets, or removing fat from your diet are ways to lose pounds, but they are only quick fixes and are not likely to last long.

In order to achieve any permanent changes, you must break down your general goals into smaller, more specific ones. You must also be aware of your habits and environment to determine whether your objectives are realistic or not. For example, if you wish to lose 15 pounds in the two weeks during Christmas break, when almost every day is a day of feasting, then chances are that you are going to have a hard time sticking to your goal.

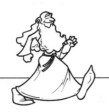

Wise Walkers

Choose a time when workload and social obligations are at a minimum. You might want to even schedule a vacation at the start of your exercise and weight-loss program to give you the feeling of a "fresh start."

For this reason, it is important for you to examine your lifestyle. Try to be honest. Pinpoint those times in the day or week when you are more susceptible to overeating. Try to determine whether these times are related to some other stressful event going on in your life. For example, do you tend to overeat when you come home after a busy day at work? Do you use food as a way to calm your nerves? Also, take a closer look at the reasons why exercise continues to drop out of your schedule only two to three weeks after beginning your program. Is there any one factor that keeps you from following through? Is it that you can never seem to get past the month mark? What happens just before you do pass that mark?

Perhaps the way you constructed your goals was inefficient the last time around and perhaps the times before that. If you continue to repeat the same patterns by setting up the same goals and approaching them the same way, then chances are that you are going to continue to fail. Perhaps it's not that you lack willpower and strength, but that you have not learned how to approach your goals effectively.

Just listing goals without taking the factors of your lifestyle into consideration is risky. You must set your goals so that they fit into your way of life. You should re-move and work around obstacles that continually get in the way of your following through with your objectives. Things don't just "happen" because you want them to. And habits don't just "go away" effortlessly without replacing them with something else. You must exchange the bad behavior with a more positive course of action in order for your efforts to stick.

Start out by listing all the reasons that contribute to keeping the weight on. Go through your daily routine and pinpoint all the problem areas that feed into (sorry) your habit of overeating. Grab your notebook and draw three lines down the page. Title the first column "Habits That Need Changing," the middle column "Alternatives," and the last column "Rewards." Make a list of all the habits to which you've attributed your weight gain in the left-hand column.

Next, take one "problem" at a time and decide how you are going to approach the situation to change it. List the solutions in the middle column of your notebook, opposite the bad habit you are focusing on. For example, if eating dessert after dinner is your problem, try to come up with a way to occupy yourself during that time, perhaps with a walk or a movie, for example, and write it down in the space opposite. If the free candy bars at work are just too tempting and you find yourself stopping by the lunchroom every hour to pick one up, prepare by bringing your own healthier snacks. Finally, make a list of all the nice things that you would like to do for yourself as a reward for your efforts. Smaller rewards should go with easier challenges. Likewise, heftier treats should be allotted for more rigorous achievements. Be reasonable. Emptying out your life savings to buy the 60-foot sailboat that you've had your eye on for the last two years, just because you skipped dessert last night, is not an equitable exchange.

Once you've completed your list, prioritize your goals. Start with the behaviors that will be least challenging to modify, and put them at the top of the page. It's better to start with smaller, more obtainable, goals in order to build your confidence. Tackling the more difficult habits first is a sure way to set yourself up for frustration and failure. Give yourself three weeks for each habit listed. In addition to writing down what you'd like to change, write down all the minor and major obstacles that might interfere with your attempts. Planning ahead of time will reduce the risk of being caught off-guard by some unforeseeable obstacle.

Wise Walkers

Choose a private time to start this list where interruptions and disturbances are not going to occur. You will really need the space and quiet to think carefully about the less-obvious habits and patterns you have incurred over time.

Keeping a Log

Keeping a log, or in this case a notebook, is an important aspect to the success of your program. Documenting everything in writing is a good way to keep you focused.

It is also a useful tool for indicating your more problematic areas. Try writing a little bit each day. Note how you feel, where you are in terms of your motivation, and any minor or major causes for frustration or concern. Patterns will emerge as you document your progression and setbacks. This is important information that will help you to devise a more effective approach next time. Plus, you will have those inevitable times when you will lose momentum, become disappointed, or become just plain bored with your program. You can expect these in every program. Having positive information about your progress in the past that you can refer to during these times is an important motivational, not to mention inspirational, tool.

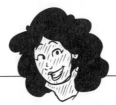

Interesting Excerpts

Many of us use food for every other reason except to satisfy hunger. Coping with stress, emotional discomfort, or a problem at work are all good examples of what I'm talking about. We're eating, but we're not really focused on what we're doing. Writing down what you eat teaches you to become a more mindful eater. A food diary can identify emotions and behaviors that trigger overeating, foster greater awareness of portion sizes, and help you discover your personal food triggers. Slowing down when you eat, tasting your food, and allowing no distractions—such as reading or watching TV—are other examples of "mindful eating."

Walkers Watch Out!

Be careful with whom you share your new plans. There are a lot of nay-sayers out there who would just love to see you fail. Seek out people who support, rather than sabotage, your efforts!

Getting and Staying Motivated

Getting motivated to start something new is one thing; staying motivated is an entirely different matter. It is easy to make grand promises to yourself, such as pledging that "this time" will be better than all the rest because "this time" is different. New Year's day, turning 30 (40, 50, 60 …), starting a new job, quitting an old job, summer vacation, breaking up with a boyfriend, meeting a new girlfriend; these are all great reasons to begin a weight-loss program.

But unless you make the commitment to yourself, for yourself, and for the right reasons, then it is going to be very difficult to stick to your promise. You must specify exactly why you would like to lose weight and get fit.

Temporary fixes to look good for your new beau is a good jump-start, but if you aren't doing it for yourself, then, chances are, it won't last.

It might help to enlist the support of a trusted friend. Perhaps, there is someone close to you, such as a co-worker or otherwise, who also wants to lose weight and get into shape. Having someone with whom you can collaborate is easier than doing it on your own. Find someone whose fitness goals are comparable to yours and who is starting from a similar place as you. Make sure your schedules are synchronized and you are equally committed to the game plan.

The Least You Need to Know

➤ Being overweight is a detriment to your health.

➤ Overcoming psychological barriers is the first hurdle toward change.

➤ Anticipating obstacles is key for a successful program.

➤ Keeping a log serves as a motivational tool.

➤ There is strength in numbers.

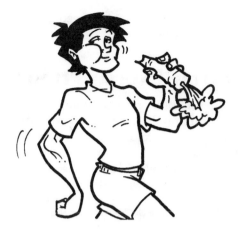

Chapter 14

Food for Thought

In This Chapter

➤ The ins and outs of weight loss

➤ Why fad diets don't work

➤ Decreasing cravings with a balanced diet

➤ Writing down what, where, and when you eat

➤ Beginning permanent weight loss with realistic goals

Trying to lose weight in America can be very confusing. There are so many different types of diets to follow, and so many mixed messages. At first there was the Pritikin and the Scarsdale diet. Next came the cabbage-soup-for-breakfast-lunch-and-dinner diet. Then we told you to cut out chewable foods altogether and to drink your meals instead. Where fat was once the culprit and carbohydrates the good guy, now carbohydrates are taking the back seat, giving you free reign to eat as much butter and mayonnaise as you want. Diet centers are paying celebrities huge amounts of money to sell *their* diets to the public. With so many conflicting messages about food and weight loss, it's no wonder that every meal has become such an anxiety-ridden experience.

Understanding how weight loss works, why the body needs certain foods, and what role exercise plays in the scheme of things are important facts to know before taking on any weight-loss challenge. In this chapter, we'll explore why and how you lose (and gain) weight. I'll show you how proper nutrition helps in stabilizing your hunger and why fad diets are dangerous. Finally, you'll get some good tips on keeping the weight off once it's been lost and how to stay focused when the going gets tough.

How Weight Loss Works and How Exercise Helps

A pound of fat equals approximately 3,500 calories. In order for you to lose (or gain) a pound, you must consume 3,500 calories less (or more) than what your body needs to perform its daily functions. The question is: How many calories does your body need? That, of course, depends on your weight and on your activity level. The heavier you are, the more calories you need to sustain your weight. If you are thinner, however, you don't have to consume as many calories to stay at your current weight. Likewise, the more energy you expend, the more calories you'll need to maintain your weight. On the other hand, if you're primarily a sedentary person with a sedentary lifestyle, you won't have to eat as much to stay the weight you are.

Wise Walkers

Two people can weigh the same amount but have totally different caloric needs depending on their activity level. The more active individual will need to consume as many as 500 calories more than his or her more sedentary counterpart just to maintain the same weight.

Eating fewer calories than what you are currently consuming will result in pounds lost. Taking in exactly 3,500 calories less than your body needs will result in a loss of one pound of body fat. But if you are only eating 2,500 calories a day, how are you going to cut your calories by 3,500? Clearly, it's impossible—which is why you can't lose a pound a day. Instead, try reducing your caloric intake by 300 to 500 a day. This could be as simple as skipping your afternoon snack of milk and cookies, or eating half instead of an entire sandwich at lunch. Over the course of a week, and if you are consistent, you will succeed in reducing your total caloric intake by 2,100 to 3,500 calories, or half a pound to a pound, which is the healthiest way to lose weight.

Walkers Watch Out!

Don't crash-diet. Experts recommend that you lose no more than one to two pounds per week. Anything more can be a risk to your health and is less likely to cause permanent weight loss.

In addition to reducing your caloric intake, you should also increase your activity level. By adding 30 to 60 minutes of activity five to seven days a week, you'll be burning 300 to 500 calories a day—or 2,100 to 3,500 calories a week—more than usual. This expenditure, combined with consuming 2,100 to 3,500 fewer calories that you're taking in through diet modifications, could reduce your total caloric intake by 4,200 to 7,000 a week, an equivalent of approximately a two-pound weight loss.

The best way to determine how many calories you are consuming currently is to keep a log of absolutely everything you eat for seven days. During this week, eat as you normally would, making no changes to your diet, since this information will tell you how many calories you're eating at your current weight, and therefore will help determine how many fewer calories you need to eat to lose weight. It is a good idea to buy a calorie counter or a book that lists food types and their caloric quantities. You can purchase these references for less than $10 at almost any bookstore. Take a look at Appendix A, "Resources for Walking Fit," for some suggestions.

At the end of each day, tally up the number of calories you've consumed. Add them up at the end of the week and divide this number by seven. Although not exact, this should give you a general number of calories you are consuming to maintain your current weight. Subtract 300 to 500 from this number; this is the maximum number of calories you need to consume to lose approximately a pound a week. I will be discussing more specific details about food choices and balancing your meals in a later section. For now, I would like you to highlight all the food items that are above and beyond your three staple meals of the day (breakfast, lunch, and dinner): I'm talking about the extras, such as afternoon snacks, sodas, and juices, the half-and-half you put in your coffee, or the bowl of ice cream after dinner. Keep this nearby, as we will be referring to it later.

Wise Walkers

You can also look online for a list of resources that will help you track what you've eaten and how many calories you've burned based on your height and weight. I found About.com's weight-loss section to be very helpful. There are sites that plan your meals for you based on your caloric requirements. There are sites that calculate the number of calories you burned doing any and all kinds of activity including vacuuming and gardening. There are sites that feature success stories of other people who've lost weight, or are trying to, who can give you advice and tips based on their experience.

Why Diets Don't Work

When people say they are on a "diet," it usually means that they have cut out certain types or amounts of food in an attempt to lose weight. Needless to say, once the weight has been lost, they return to their former style of eating and, within a month

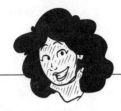

Interesting Excerpts

When you say you're on a "diet," it implies that it is only a temporary thing. When you say you are improving your eating habits, it implies a long-lasting, or even lifelong, change.

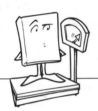

Weighty Words

Your **BMR,** or **basal metabolic rate,** is the energy expended by the body at rest to maintain normal bodily functions. This continual work makes up about 60 to 70 percent of the calories we use ("burn," or expend), and includes the beating of our heart, respiration, and the maintenance of body temperature.

or two (sometimes less), they've gained back all the weight they lost. But weight does not magically stay off once it's been lost (especially if you return to your old eating habits; you know, the ones that put the pounds on in the first place?). You must maintain a lower-calorie "diet" to maintain your "lower" weight. Remember? The lighter you are, the fewer calories you need.

Diets, per se, are just temporary fixes. Severely restricting what you can and cannot eat may cause some weight loss, but only for the time being. It is highly unlikely, no matter how much you may pride yourself on your iron will, that you'll be able to stick with anything that is too unrealistic and hard to fit into your everyday life. It is only a matter of time before you "break the rules" or "slip" from the program.

Beyond setting you up for failure, diets can also cause you to gain more weight when all is said and done. That's right, diets can make you fatter! How, you ask? Well, it works like this: Your body needs a certain amount of calories (energy) in order to perform properly. Your heart, lungs, muscles, and everything else your body is made of needs fuel, in the form of food, to function. This is what is known as your *BMR,* or *basal metabolic rate.* When it does not get enough "fuel," your metabolism slows down in an attempt to preserve that which it has. It is a survival tactic to ward off starvation.

Of course, you also will naturally lose some weight as the body sheds water and uses some of the excess fat to feed itself. Happy with the weight loss, you return to more normal eating patterns. Unbeknownst to you, however, your metabolism remains in its impeded state. It needs fewer calories to sustain itself, and you begin to gain weight without even increasing your caloric intake.

The Balancing Act: Your Basic Food Pyramid

Balance and moderation are the magic words. Ever hear the saying "all things in moderation"? Well, the same goes for food. It's neither necessary nor healthy to completely cut out entire food groups. Of course, exceptions include people who are vegetarians and choose not to eat animal meat, and people who have allergies to specific foods and must, therefore, eliminate them from their diets. But, for the most part, you should be able to enjoy any and all kinds of food "in moderation."

Walkers Watch Out!

A diet of less than 1,000 to 1,200 calories can actually cause a starvation-like state and force your body to conserve calories. The body will cut back its energy expenditure to survive. This slows down the metabolism for as long as one year. That's why so many people have difficulty losing weight after years and years of extreme dieting. Their metabolisms are all out of whack and they can't even eat "normally" without gaining weight.

The problem with Americans is not necessarily what we eat, but the fact that we eat too much. Our portions are enormous! One of our meals is comparable to two and even three meals in other countries around the world. Not only are our portions huge, but we also feel, for some reason or another, obliged to lick the plate clean at every meal. If we don't, we feel we've deprived or "cheated" ourselves. We eat until we feel full and then we eat some more.

To make matters worse, we've built fast-food establishments at every corner, and most are designed so that you don't even have to get out of the car and walk to order your food. In addition to our flourishing consumption of fast fatty foods is our declining consumption of fresh fruits and vegetables. Processed, canned, and sprayed foods rob our foods of many of the vitamins and minerals we need to function healthfully.

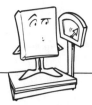

Weighty Words

Did you know that the **hypothalamus** is a part of the brain that is known for the regulation of eating? It signals to our stomach when it is full and when it is not about 10 minutes after digestion has begun.

Furthermore, because you are not getting the nutrients you need, your appetite is never really satisfied. For example, you may find that you always feel hungry or crave "something," but you don't know what. This is your body's way of telling you it needs more nutrients. Unfortunately, rather than eating more of the right thing, you eat more of the wrong, which only exacerbates the problem even further.

Walkers Watch Out!

Avoid fast food whenever possible. Did you know that 360 of the 660 total calories of a Burger King Whopper come from fat? That means that more than half of the total calories are fat calories.

For these reasons, it is imperative that you develop a balanced and well-rounded (no pun intended) diet. Eating a moderate amount of a variety of foods will ensure that you are not only getting the nutrients you need but are also satisfying your appetite, to avoid cravings and the possibility of maluntrition.

In 1992, the Food and Drug Administration (FDA) came up with the concept of the Food Pyramid. The Food Pyramid is exactly that: a pyramid whose triangular shape corresponds to the quantity of servings we should consume from each layer of the pyramid. In other words, those foods at the wider portion of the pyramid should make up the majority of our diet, while those foods at the top should comprise the least part of our diet. Following is an illustration of the food pyramid.

At the base, you have your grains: pasta, rice, bread, crackers, cereals. You should eat six to eleven servings from this group. The next layer is fruits (two to four servings) and vegetables (three to five servings). Farther up the triangle are meat and dairy products. You should consume two to three servings of each daily. Finally, at the top, the smallest portion of the triangle, are your sweets, fats, and oils, of which you should use sparingly.

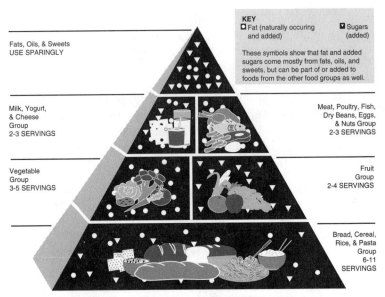

Source: U.S. Department of Agriculture - U.S. Department of Health and Human Services

Wise Walkers

Cravings are said to be the body's way of telling you that it's lacking a particular nutrient. If you've been on a severely restrictive diet, or you do not vary the types of food you eat on a regular basis, then perhaps your cravings are trying to tell you something.

A "serving" is not simply a plop of mashed potatoes or several large slices of roast beef. A "serving" as defined by the FDA is comprised of a very specific amount of food. For example, six to eleven servings of grains may sound like a lot, but when you consider the actual amount of each serving, it is easy to see how one could fill their daily requirements in two sittings (or even one). The following table gives a guideline for "servings."

Food Group	Type	Amount
Grains	bread	1 slice
	pasta	$1/2$ cup cooked
	rice	$1/2$ cup cooked
	cereal	1 ounce
Vegetables	green leafy	1 cup raw
	carrots	$1/2$ cup
	broccoli	1 cup
Fruits	apple	1 medium
	berries	$1/2$ cup
	banana	1 medium
Proteins	meat/poultry	2 to 3 ounces
	fish	2 to 3 ounces
	egg	1
	nuts	2 tbsp.
Fats and oils		use sparingly
	butter	use sparingly
Sweets	candy	use sparingly

It is unlikely that you will gain weight if you follow these pyramid guidelines. In fact, altering your diet to include the specifications above will most likely lead to some weight loss initially, both because you'll be eating healthier food (probably), but also because you'll be eating less.

Changing Habits and Lifestyle

Now that we've got all the details about the types and amounts of food you should be eating, let's discuss how you are going to adapt this to fit into your current lifestyle. You'll remember in Chapter 13, "Weight Walkers," we discussed the importance of re-defining your goals. I had you write down all of your "bad" habits and how you plan to change them, remember? Now let's explore how you are going to ease these healthier food choices into your diet.

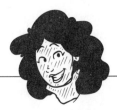

Interesting Excerpts

Substantial change is not something that comes easily. In order for change to stick, you must allow your body and your mind to acclimate to the shift. Altering a bunch of deeply ingrained behavioral patterns all at once only serves to overwhelm the psyche, which inevitably leads to confusion and failure.

With your notebook in hand, flip to the section where you recorded your weekly caloric intake. Review the items you highlighted again. With the food pyramid in mind, take a closer look at some other modifications you can make to improve your diet. Analyze your meals according to the guidelines set up by the pyramid. This way you will be able to see more clearly those areas that need more help than others.

Rather than substituting something at every meal, start by making exchanges one by one. For example, cut down on your butter for several weeks. Don't worry about anything else, just your butter intake. When you feel confident that you've adjusted to this change, move on to your dairy products. Replace whole milks and yogurts with skim or low-fat. Every time you succeed at changing something, reward yourself. Don't be too hard on yourself; this is a lifestyle change, so you've got some time to make a few mistakes here and there. Remember to keep it simple.

One Day at a Time

Last, but certainly not least, is the importance of maintaining perspective. Getting too caught up and consumed with weight loss, diet, exercise, calories, or fat percentages can take up a lot of time, not to mention money. Besides, you should have better things to do with your days. Assuming that you have "the rest of your life" to live, it is a good idea not to take everything so seriously. Define your goals, set up your plan, make your commitment, and then get out there and enjoy life a little. After all, the less pressure you put on yourself, the more likely you are to succeed at making permanent lifestyle changes rather than just temporary fixes.

The Least You Need to Know

➤ The more activities you perform, the more calories you expend.

➤ Diets that are too impractical are often unsuccessful.

➤ A well-balanced diet helps to satisfy the appetite.

➤ Changing habits one at a time is better than tackling them all at once.

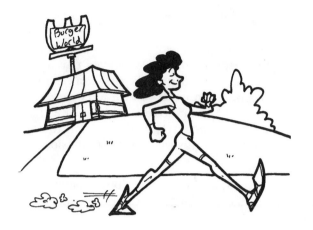

Chapter 15

Fast Feet, Not Fast Food

In This Chapter

➤ Why you gain and lose weight

➤ Using walking to increase your metabolism

➤ What speed and hills have in common

➤ Understanding the pain factor

➤ Finding a place for plateaus

Talking the talk is one thing; walking the walk is quite another. Up to this point, we've explored some of the issues behind noncompliance, weight loss and gain, and changing old behavioral patterns. We've discovered a new way to view the "four food groups," and you now know that "diets don't work," and that in order for you to lose weight you must cut back on your caloric intake while increasing your activity level. At this point, you are probably feeling pretty on the ball about the whole weight thing.

In this chapter, I'll provide you with some suggestions about planning your course of action to ensure a safe and long-lasting change. I will talk about the possibility of having feelings of discomfort and how to overcome them. I will also give you some ideas on when and how to adjust the intensity of your walks to keep your body challenged. Finally, you will discover ways to vary your routine to avoid boredom so that you may enjoy walking for months and years to come.

Understanding the Nature of Caloric Expenditure

In Chapter 14, "Food for Thought," I reviewed the Basal Metabolic Rate—the minimum number of calories your body needs to function properly. When you have exceeded this "necessary" amount of energy intake, your body stores the extra calories (energy) in the form of fat. This is why you gain weight when you eat too much. Similarly, when you are not consuming a sufficient amount of food, or if your activity level supersedes the amount of calories you've consumed, your body will start to use the "stored" fuel and you will begin to lose weight. This is what health professionals call the *energy balance equation*.

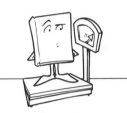

Weighty Words

The **energy balance equation** means that to lose weight, you must consume fewer calories than you burn—or, in reverse, you must burn more calories than you consume.

This equation includes a negative caloric balance and a positive caloric balance. Negative caloric balance means that you expend more calories than the amount of calories your body requires to sustain its current weight. The result is weight loss. A positive caloric balance means that you are consuming more calories than your body needs to sustain its current weight (you got it: weight gain). The aim, of course, is to equalize the amount of energy that comes in (via food) with the amount of energy that goes out (activity, basal metabolic functioning) once you've reached your goal weight. But first you must reach your goal weight.

You can achieve weight loss in two ways: You can cut your caloric intake (which we've discussed in previous chapters) or you can increase the number of calories you expend with exercise (which is what we'll talk about here).

Pacing Yourself

Knowing how much to exercise is key. Too much too soon can (and often does) lead to program drop-out. Chances are that you have been pretty inactive lately. Sure, you may walk to the corner store or walk to and from the subway station five days a week, but beyond that, your muscles, heart, and lungs have been pretty dormant, right? If this sounds familiar, make sure that you pay extra attention to pacing yourself and taking it slow in the beginning.

Frequency First

Obviously, the more you exercise, the more calories you burn. But because your body is not used to moving for extended periods of time, it is unwise to set you loose for several hours all at once. Instead, it's better to start with a short amount of time, and to increase the number of days you exercise instead. Walking more days for shorter periods of time is easier on your body than walking more time for fewer days. Compare it to cramming for a test three days before the exam versus learning a little bit each day for a month. Chances are that the latter will have you walking away not only with more knowledge retained, but also a lot less tired as well.

Start off with just a few minutes, three days a week. Try to get out at lunchtime or after dinner for a 5- to 10-minute walk around the neighborhood. Don't worry about how fast you're going, or whether you're "feeling" it or not—that's not the point right now. Remember that you're trying to get your body used to an increase in activity while training your mind to carve out this time into your weekly routine. When you're ready, add another day until you are walking at least every other day.

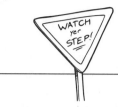

Walkers Watch Out!

Don't panic if you're hungry! Some people experience a rise in appetite with the onset of exercise. This is normal and to be expected. Work around your appetite by planning your meals ahead of time rather than eating impulsively.

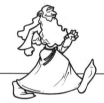

Wise Walkers

Emphasizing frequency first helps to build the "habit" of exercise into your daily routine. Habits are just patterns of behavior that we learn. Increasing the amount you walk establishes routine and patterns into your daily agenda. It doesn't matter so much how long or how far but how often you walk. Soon you will expect rather than remind yourself that today is your day for walking without giving it a second thought, and walking will become just another habit.

Adding Time

Once you've worked up to 5 to 15 minutes of walking "most" days of the week, you can start increasing the time (in the form of minutes) of each of your daily walks. Add five minutes to each day that you walk. Give yourself a week in between to allow your body to adjust then add another five minutes. Keep doing this until you feel you've reached your goal or time limit.

Intensity Last

Of course, there are only so many days in the week and so many minutes in the day, right? At some point our lives will interfere and we'll have to get back to work, the kids, visiting friends—other activities not related to exercise, right? If you've added as much time as your schedule allows, and you are walking as many days as you can manage without being accused of abandoning your family, the next step you'll need to make is to adjust the intensity of your walks. Increasing the intensity and *power* of your workouts enables you to get as much (and often more) work in the same (if not less) amount of time. Plus, high-intensity walks are a great way to save time.

So, why didn't I just skip to this part from the beginning? Well, because if I had, chances are that you would have injured yourself and would be unable to make it past the first week. The reason why higher-intensity walks are so efficient is because they challenge your body at least twice as much as "normal" walking does. But to do so, your body needs to be in that much better condition to accommodate the challenge, as well as needing that much more time to recover.

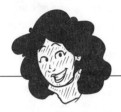

Interesting Excerpts

Power walking is simply very fast walking and can, some believe, burn more calories than running. A competitive power walker can walk a marathon, 26.2 miles, from 5$^1/_2$ to 8 hours. A pedometer measures the length of the power walkers stride to figure how many miles are being walked.

With this in mind, it is imperative that you take extra care when you increase the intensity of your weekly walks. It is not necessary, nor advised, to walk at a high intensity every day. Try adding one day of increased intensity every two weeks. Because you are putting more stress and strain on your body, it will naturally need more time to recover. After two to three weeks have passed, add another day. Try to balance your "harder" days with your "easier" days. Generally speaking, your walking routine should be comprised of no more that 30 percent of higher-intensity walks. Spread them out, since your body will need time to recuperate from the added strain you've put on it.

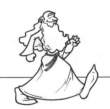

Wise Walkers

Increasing intensity is not limited to modifying your speed. You can make your walks harder by walking hills, carrying weights, changing your terrain, carrying a backpack, or just altering your stride.

In terms of your heart rate, you should keep it somewhere between 75 to 85 percent of your max for your higher-intensity walking days. If you are unable to maintain this level for 30 minutes at a time, then do it in bouts. For example, after a 10-minute warm-up at 60 to 65 percent of your max, bring your heart rate up a few notches to 70 to 75 percent for the next 5 minutes, and then up to 80 to 85 percent for the following 5 minutes after that. See how this feels at this higher level. Bring it back down to 75 to 80 percent for 5 minutes just to give your heart a rest. Repeat this cycle four times if you are walking for 20 minutes, five times for 25, six times for 30, and so on. Refer to Chapter 2, "One Step at a Time," for examples of age-predicted heart-rate maximums and subsequent percentages thereof.

Suggestion for Adjusting Intensity

The most obvious way to adjust intensity is to walk faster. For most of you, however, there is a limit to how fast you can walk. No matter how hard you try, you just can't make your legs move any quicker. Yet you want to up the ante. You know you are in better shape. You can feel it. Activities that once seemed difficult and laborious have become easier and more enjoyable. So, what's next? How can you challenge yourself without having to break into a trot? Following is a list that reviews ways you can make your walking workout harder, including some modifications you should be aware of if you are carrying around a lot of weight.

➤ **Beach walking** (Chapter 6): If you are carrying a lot of extra weight, make sure that you take it slow. Walking on sand already puts additional strain on your joints.

➤ **Walking hills** (Chapter 6): Walking downhill can put added stress on your lower back and knees, so make sure you take it slow by taking small, light strides. Try not to walk hills more than two times a week, and spread the days out so that you give your body a rest in between.

➤ **Water walking:** Water offers a safe mode of resistance, and it can be very effective for burning extra calories. In fact, you can burn over 600 calories an hour walking through water. It is also much easier on your bones. Water is denser than air and is therefore more buoyant, releasing some of the weight from your joints.

Walkers Watch Out!

Pushing your body past its comfort zone means that you are adding excess stress to your immune system. Save higher-intensity workouts for when you are good and healthy. Avoid doing them after recovering from an illness like the flu or a cold.

Wise Walkers

The Aquatic Exercise Association is a nonprofit organization committed to increasing the healthy life span for individuals through education and participation in safe and effective aquatic exercise programs. You can reach them at: PO Box 1609, Nokomis, FL 34274-1609, 1-888-AEA-WAVE (toll-free), or 941-486-8600.

Walking Through the Discomfort

Starting anything new will inevitably bring some discomfort, both physically and mentally. Chances are that you have been relatively inactive of late, so any kind of stress on your system is going to result in some pain and soreness. This is to be expected. Soreness is just the body's way of telling you that you've pushed it beyond its comfort level. Fortunately, our bodies are very adaptable organisms. Excess stress stimulates growth, so eventually that which seemed hard becomes easier.

Acute or prolonged pain is not normal, however. If you've been experiencing extreme discomfort or sharp, piercing pain anywhere in or on your body, then there is a chance that something more serious is going on. If this is the case, stop exercising and make an appointment with your health professional. If it feels unhealthy, then it probably is.

You might also experience some emotional discomfort when you first start exercising. We discussed some reasons behind this in the "Psychological Barriers and Social Shyness" section of Chapter 13, "Weight Walkers." Remember that every beginner (no matter what activity it is) experiences some uneasiness and awkwardness. That which does not come naturally will present a challenge to your comfort level. Like the body, the mind will also grow stronger once the challenge has been met, however. Experience breeds confidence, but you must have the courage and the tenacity to stick with it first.

Postulating Plateaus

Have you ever reached a point in your exercise career when, no matter how much you've stuck to the plan, you can't seem to get any stronger or drop any more weight? Your progress seems to have just leveled off, and try as you may, you just can't figure out what has gone wrong? Everybody reaches *plateaus* at some (many) points in his or her exercise and diet career. A plateau is your body's way of telling you that it needs to be challenged in a different way, or that it just needs a little break. As you know, your system adjusts to excess stress and strain by becoming stronger. As you continue to overload it, the body will continue to accommodate the challenge by becoming more efficient. Once the body has become efficient at an activity, however, it will return to a less-heightened state of stimulation. It will adapt to the stress of a new activity and become more proficient at performing it.

Similarly, as you lose weight, your body will expend fewer calories at the same activity level. In other words, the lighter you are, the harder you will have to work if you want to burn the same amount of calories that you burned 15 pounds heavier. A 150-pound woman expends more calories walking the same route for one hour than a 130-pound woman does, for instance. This is because she has more mass to carry through space. Her muscles, bones, lungs, and heart have to work harder to accommodate the weight of the extra 20 pounds.

It is very common, therefore, to hear "dieters" complain that despite their diligence and commitment to stick to their plan, they can't seem to drop any more weight. They've lost the first 15 pounds but just cannot get rid of the last 5.

When you reach such a plateau, you'll have to adjust either the intensity of your walks or your caloric intake. Because you weigh less, your body requires fewer calories to sustain its current weight. In other words, your BMR has decreased. The negative caloric balance from the beginning of your program has leveled off due to the change in your body weight.

If you want to lose more weight, you will either have to reduce your caloric intake even more so that the "balance" becomes negative again, or increase the intensity of your caloric expenditure. For example, you might substitute one of your flat days with another hill day. You could also add 10 minutes to each of your walks, or pick up the pace a little. If restricting your caloric intake seems like torture and fills you with dread, then perhaps you should opt for the second choice and up the ante of your walking routine instead.

You Win Sum and You Lose Sum: A Summary

You can buy weight-loss pills, diet books, exercise equipment, and even surgery to "fix" your weight problem. But these are temporary and sometimes dangerous options. The best way to ensure healthy weight loss is through exercise and diet modification. Gradually replacing your poor eating habits with better ones will promote more lasting change. Walking is an excellent form of exercise since it is both efficient and safe, but any type of movement (as long as it's more than what you are doing now) is going to help you lose weight and keep it off, as well as improve your health.

Perhaps the most important lesson to take away from the last three chapters is that you must be patient. Remember that you are making a lifestyle change. You are altering behavioral patterns that have been a part of who you are for years. Anytime you get distracted by a promise that sounds "too good to be true," remind yourself that it probably is. Substantial change takes time and is usually most successful by taking small steps at a time.

Stay away from the media (magazines, TV, movies) for a while if you can. Work on changing your self-image from within rather than getting caught up in the extreme stereotypes of external beauty our culture displays. Try to put your well-being, rather than your vanity, first. It will make it a lot easier to persevere when you realize your health is on the line.

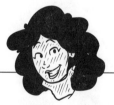

Interesting Excerpts

To borrow the words from E. J. Green, Ph.D.: "Preferably, change is gradual and orderly, old behaviors slowly giving way to new and more useful ones, until a new balance is struck."

The Least You Need to Know

➤ You must expend more calories than you take in if you want to lose weight.

➤ Shorter bouts of walking are best when starting a program.

➤ Intensity should be the last adjustment you make to your program.

➤ Slight discomfort and mild soreness are to be expected when you begin any new activity.

➤ You must continually challenge your system if you want it to change.

Part 4

Walking as a Lifestyle

So, you've reached your goals. You've lost those extra 15 pounds, your doctor says your blood pressure has dropped, and you are able to walk five miles without having to take a breather. Now you're ready to stop. You've done your dirty work, right?

Wrong! Walking is a lifestyle. All those good things you worked so hard to achieve will slowly start to backslide if you don't keep up the work. Remember: "Use it or lose it." One of the hardest concepts for people to accept is that walking, and exercise in general, is a lifelong endeavor. Here, in this part, I'll show you how to incorporate walking into your everyday life as well as some tricks and tips for avoiding excuses and drop-out. I'll also give you some suggestions for walking in different kinds of weather, and how to use the gym and your home to best suit your walking needs.

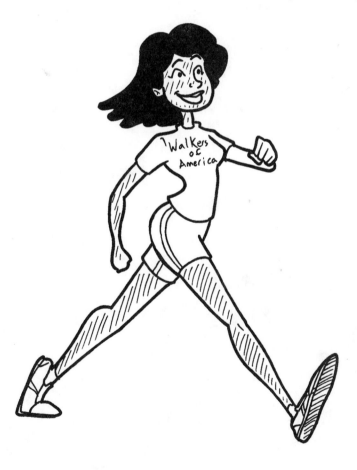

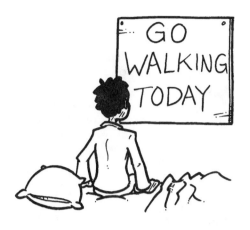

Chapter 16

Waste Not, Walk Not

In This Chapter

➤ The danger of the excuse

➤ Making realistic choices

➤ Substituting good habits for bad ones

➤ How to handle "slips"

You all know how easy it is to become excited about the idea of becoming someone new? Admit it, it's fun to fantasize about how glamorous and different everything will be once you've become the "improved you." TV, magazines, movies, and the Internet only serve to encourage this way of thinking. Images of beautiful people (cosmetic surgery, computer enhancing, lighting, and *lots* of makeup) with perfect lives (studio sets) litter the airways 24 hours a day, seven days a week, sending the message that we are imperfect and need to change—immediately—to make us better people.

Unfortunately, what the media neglects to tell you is that in order to make any significant changes, you need to work hard and you need to have patience (and, unfortunately, patience does not sell). No, you prefer the "quick fix," the miraculous transition from A to B, and without immediate results you are ready to give up without even trying. Frustration, feelings of failure, and low self-esteem serve only to exacerbate the problem of "imperfection" even further.

Reaching your goals is not an impossible task, but it is possible only if you are patient enough to follow the steps that are involved in getting there. You wouldn't build a house without first establishing a sturdy foundation, would you? Well, the same goes for your goals. In order for them to be substantial you must take the steps to make them so. That's what we'll discuss in this chapter.

No Excuses!

Merriam-Webster's Dictionary defines "option" as an "act of choosing, the power or right to choose" or "freedom of choice." It is this "choice" that you must consider carefully before you take on any serious commitment. You must realize all of the implications, the gains, and the losses, that each choice involves. Once you have taken the time to review these, then you must move forward with the decision of which "choice" to make without looking back.

Making a pledge to walk, and to health, is a choice. Once you've made the choice to improve your well-being, and you've defined how you plan to do it, it should be nonnegotiable. Making the decision in the first place implies that you've reviewed all of the obstacles that could get in your way and that you have devised ways around them. Once you've reached this point, excuses should be banned entirely.

Excuses are basically justifications for not following through with your commitment to yourself or to someone else. But whatever you tell yourself and others, you know deep inside that you are letting yourself down. You are compromising your confidence and going back on the promise you made for your own good. Years of excuses could lower your self-confidence and leave you feeling pretty darn bad, making it all that much harder to attempt such challenges in the future.

You must attempt to keep the excitement and the passion that you started with close at hand. You will inevitably have times during your program when you are tired, bored, or just plain lazy. The fantasy of the "new you" has evolved into something a little more real and it's not exactly what you had in mind. It is during these times that you ought to rely on the memory of your initial enthusiasm, and to remember your promise to yourself and why you began this quest in the first place. You know the saying, "when the going gets tough, the tough get going"? Well, it's during these "tough" times that your real strength shines through.

Daily Reminders

An effective way to keep the enthusiasm alive is through daily reminders. Small things like inspirational quotes, notes to yourself, and encouraging photographs posted in areas visible to the eye act to remind you of why you initially decided to make this commitment to yourself. Getting caught up in the hustle and bustle of everyday life has a very tricky way of distracting you from your goals. It is easier to rely on old patterns during times of stress and chaos. It's what is familiar and comfortable to you. New habits don't stick that easily in the beginning, so you must remind yourself to see them through. Posting little notes and photographs everywhere around your home, car, and office helps you to catch yourself in the midst of repeating old habits and patterns.

Inspirational Images

Nothing works better to encourage you than a photo of someone you admire. What's the saying? "A picture speaks a thousand words"? Having a photograph of your mentor, someone you know (or not) who has succeeded in doing what you have set out to do, is a great way to stay focused. Make sure you choose a person who shares similar goals and aspirations to yours. It's best to choose someone you can relate to, whose life resembles your life, in order to make your goals seem that much more obtainable. Posting photographs of pre-pubescent male supermodels around your office might be a little inappropriate if you are a 45-year-old man looking for inspiration to start a walking program.

Wise Walkers

Spend a few minutes each night creating a new inspirational reminder for yourself. This will not only add some fun to the process, but it will also act as an extra reminder in itself.

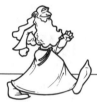

Wise Walkers

I suggest flipping through the fitness magazines at your local grocery store. Many issues feature real life "success stories" of individuals who have attained the very goals you are setting out to achieve. They are good, practical images to keep alive in your memory during those tougher times. You can also check online resources for interactive chats and support groups. There are many people out there who are on the same quest as you and they are more than happy to exchange ideas, tips, and personal experience. Keep these Web sites in your personal favorites so that you have quick and easy access to them when your confidence dwindles.

Noticeable Notes

Another excellent way to remind yourself of your goals is to post little notes for yourself everywhere. I know, I know: It probably sounds a little neurotic and obsessive, right? What would your family think? Doesn't matter what they think, because it works. Like I mentioned earlier, it is very easy to get side-tracked and distracted by the rigmarole of life. Having little notes strategically placed throughout your home and office helps to bring your attention back to the larger picture that is your commitment to a healthier, happier life.

Imagine coming home from a busy day at the office. Despite the fact that you've made promise upon promise to yourself that you will go for a walk after work, all you really want to do is sit down and veg out in front of the TV. How do you think you would feel picking up a remote control that had a note with the message "Put me down and go for a walk" stuck on it? How easy would it be to ignore the note posted on the TV screen instructing you to: "Turn me off. Remember your promise"? How about opening the refrigerator to a note that reads: "A walk a day keeps the pounds away?"

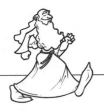

Wise Walkers

Buy an assortment of different colored post-its, the brighter the better. Frequently rewrite the same notes on different colors of post-its so the message remains fresh in your brain.

Try to make the message humorous with a touch of seriousness. You don't need to reprimand yourself at every turn. Place these notes in areas where you are most likely to find yourself during the times that you originally set aside for exercise. If you normally end up in the kitchen rather than in the gym, put a note on the kitchen table, in the cupboards, or outside the refrigerator door. If you always end up on the phone rather than on the track, place a note around the receiver or on the table by the phone. Catch yourself before you've gone home by placing notes at work or in your car. This way you can turn your car around and head straight for the trails before it's too late.

Supportive Situations

Surrounding yourself with supportive people is another very important factor in successfully obtaining your goals. People who believe in what you're doing, and who can provide motivation when yours is dwindling, are a resource not to be ignored. I have had many times when one of my sisters has encouraged me to take my training to a level I didn't think was possible. Despite my own doubts, they believed in me and encouraged me to try harder. Or, at other times I didn't feel like working out, but I had to because I had made a date with a friend several weeks earlier—one that we "promised" not to break.

Breaking commitments to yourself is a lot easier than breaking commitments to other people. Appointments—time and energy spent in collaboration with someone else—involve a level of expectancy and pressure that you might not uphold for yourself. Choose someone you trust. Make sure that they are looking after you and not trying to sabotage your program. Success can ignite jealousy and envy in others, especially in those who have not been successful at their own attempts, so make sure you stay clear of these types. Try to pick people to whom you have not previously made failed promises. Even though they may be happy to provide their support, a reminder of your failure will remain alive in your memory every time you see them. Finally, limit the number of people you commit to. Some pressure is okay, but overdoing it by telling the entire office or extended family can be too much to bear.

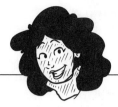

Interesting Excerpts

There are literally thousands of walking groups and clubs in the United States and internationally. The IW is the largest walking club organization in the world, with thousands of member clubs, including over 500 in the United States and Canada. Joining a walking group is an excellent way to tap into support. Not only will you be meeting people with similar goals to yours, you'll also remain somewhat anonymous, making it easier to rebuild the image of the "new" you. You can find resources for walking groups online, at your local health club, or through your medical center, as many of these places are sponsors for walking groups.

Writing Walking into Your Schedule

We've discussed the importance of carving out time in your calendar for new activities. Simply saying that you will walk "when you have time" is never going to work, as the distractions of the day will inevitably fill your time without an ounce to spare. If you want to succeed at starting and maintaining a walking habit, you must be proactive and block out the time in your schedule. Otherwise, it just won't happen. So, drag out the calendar again and let's take a closer look.

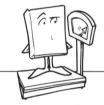

If you know that you want to commit to four days of walking a week, start by choosing those days that are easiest to manipulate timewise. For most people this would mean *weekends*. Find an hour during both Saturday and Sunday when you will be able to get away from the "errands" and distractions of the day for your weekly walk. For some people, this may be early mornings while the kids are still sleeping. Others might choose the lazy part of the day between lunch and dinner. You could also schedule errands in with your daily dose of exercise by walking to the grocery store, the dry cleaners, and the barber. Whatever the time, choose it ahead of time and black it out with permanent ink.

Weighty Words

Weekend doesn't necessarily have to mean Saturday and Sunday. When I say weekend, I am basically referring to your days off from work. This could be a day or two in the middle of the week for some of you.

Now that we've taken care of two out of the four days, let's take a closer look at the rest of your week. Finding an hour during the workweek can be quite a challenge for many of you, especially since more and more people are so busy that they don't even have time to take a lunch break. Needless to say, this is not good. Being too busy to eat can be counterproductive to meeting your goals, not to mention detrimental to your health. If you're an extremely busy person, you must be creative when it comes to finding time in your crazy day for yourself. The following are some suggestions that might be useful:

➤ Walk to work.

➤ Park as far as you can from the office and walk the distance.

➤ Make an appointment with yourself. Have your assistant write a name in the hour-long slot to trick you into not canceling at the last minute.

➤ Take your workout clothes with you to work and go for a walk before heading home.

➤ Get up a little earlier and walk before work begins.

➤ Suggest a walk rather than lunch for an employee meeting.

Reserve the time in your schedule at least two to four weeks ahead of time. This way you can anticipate obstacles and plan around them. Be flexible when you need to be. Don't try to set up too strict of a program since it will inevitably end up being too hard to keep. And remember that fitness is a way of life, so it must "fit in" to your way of life if it's going to work out in the long run.

Keeping Your Gear Handy

Being prepared is another way to avoid excuses and last-minute cancellations. Having everything you need within close proximity enables you to be more flexible with your time. Having to rush home to get your workout gear introduces the temptation of interruptions and distractions. If you have your gym bag in the trunk of your car or at work, then you can avoid the lure of "flaking out on the couch," and you can get your workout out of the way before you go home.

Try to make it as easy as possible for yourself. The more complicated it is, the less likely it is to last. Not having to think about the possibility of distractions and interruptions will make sticking to your program even easier. Treat yourself to a new wardrobe of walking and workout gear. Buy an extra gym bag, fill it with your new gear, and stick it in the back of your car. During the day, you can leave it in your trunk or

Walkers Watch Out!

Don't forget your shoes! Always have an extra pair of shoes, one for home and one for work. That way if you leave the pair at work, you won't have an excuse not to walk on the weekends.

take it into the office with you. Place one of your "noticeable" notes on the dashboard and on your desk to remind yourself that you've made a commitment to stop by the track or the gym for a three-mile walk before going home. Change at work if you have to.

Changing Habits One Step at a Time

I've discussed (over and over and over again) the importance of gradual change versus quick fixes. If you expect to make any long-term changes, they need to be tackled one at a time. The reason for this is simple. A habit is, according to the *Merriam-Webster Dictionary* definition, an "acquired mode of behavior that has become nearly or completely involuntary." Thus, because habits are involuntary, you can perform bad habits without really noticing them, unless you work hard to increase your awareness of them. If you attempt to change more than one habit at a time, chances are that you will neglect one as you make painstaking efforts to remember the other. It's only a matter of time before you're left feeling stressed and completely overwhelmed.

Take a moment and think about the habits you'd like to change. Write down anything and everything that comes to mind; just let your imagination run wild. When you've completed the list, review it. Cross off anything that is unrealistic. Your challenges should be achievable and within the realm of possibility. If goals are not attainable, then cross them out. Next, try to put them in order of importance. For example, if quitting smoking is one of the habits you'd like to change, but you'd also like to become more active, try to decide which one is more important. Spend some time prioritizing your list.

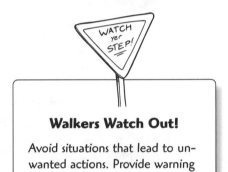

Walkers Watch Out!

Avoid situations that lead to unwanted actions. Provide warning signs. Break the chain early.

Once you've completed this list, draw a line down the center of the page and write a substitute behavior for each habit you would like to change. For example, a substitute behavior for smoking might be popping a piece of gum in your mouth every time you feel the need for a cigarette. The alternatives should be relatively simple and attainable. Write a date next to each substitute. Be careful not to be overly ambitious. Give yourself enough time to adjust to the new behavior before moving on to another one.

Finally, draw a third line down the page and list the treats you will reward yourself with every time you successfully replace a bad habit with a good one. The magnitude of the reward should be proportionate to the size of the achievement. Buying yourself a new car just for taking the stairs that day is an example of a disproportionate reward. Last, be sure to take the time to congratulate yourself on your success. You deserve it. You've worked hard and made some sacrifices. Now you are entitled to enjoy the glory of victory.

177

Staying Focused

Staying focused is not an easy job, especially when the stresses of the day take over. That's why it's important to have visible and accessible reminders within eyesight to remain focused on your goals. In addition to reminders, making your transition from a "bad" habit to a more positive one should be made as easy and simple as possible. Being overwhelmed by complicated "rules and regulations" is sure to overwhelm you and jeopardize your efforts.

In addition to the preceding suggestions, you might want to find a way to remind yourself of the consequences of returning to your old habits. Write down something about a difficult moment you had before you started to exercise. Pin up a photo of yourself at a time when you were less pleased with your appearance or your health. Post the results of your cholesterol test on the refrigerator door. Whatever it may be, keep the consequences of *relapse* close at hand.

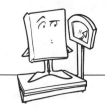

Weighty Words

Relapse is the act or an instance of backsliding, worsening, or subsiding.

If you do end up taking a couple of steps back, don't sweat it. After all, you're human and humans do make mistakes. If you are too hard on yourself, you will probably end up having expectations that are too high and too difficult to attain. When you don't do what you've set out to do for the day, just tell yourself that you'll "let it go" this time. Spending too much energy on berating yourself will only serve to lower your confidence, which increases your chances of "failure" even more. Focus on recommitting rather than omitting your goals. Review the inspirational images and noticeable notes you posted around the house and your office, or just create some more. Get yourself in a positive frame of mind rather than wasting time getting down on yourself.

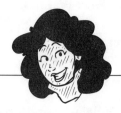

Interesting Excerpts

Clinical psychologist Clayton Tucker-Ladd suggests "self-testing in fantasy how well you would handle several high-risk situations" and "observing your lapse and relapse fantasies or temptations; i.e., imagine how you might relapse" in order to prepare yourself to handle the worst.

Stay away from situations that trigger old behaviors. If you've never been able to get to the gym after arriving home from work, then don't go home first. Bring your workout clothes with you so you can stop by the gym before going home. If you always overeat when you go out for lunch, bring your own lunch instead. It may feel a little awkward not to join the gang for lunch, but only at first. Explain your reasons for not going and ask for their support. Be extra attentive during high-stress and overly emotive periods, since these are the times when most people revert to their old habits.

The Least You Need to Know

➤ Fast changes are just quick and temporary fixes.

➤ Keeping consequences close at hand is a strong motivator.

➤ The best way to let go of old habits is to replace them with new ones.

➤ Rewarding your successes leads to more success.

➤ Staying focused takes self-discipline and control.

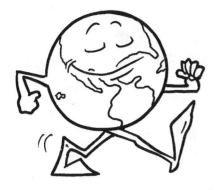

Chapter 17

This Is a Walking World

In This Chapter

➤ Finding ways to incorporate more walking into your day

➤ Making every little bit count

➤ Walking after dinner to help digestion

➤ Using the pup to pick up the pace

➤ How shopping can get you into shape

The beauty of walking is that you can do it practically anywhere and everywhere. Whether you are going to and from work, traveling, shopping, running an errand, or just hanging out with a friend, walking can be added to your day no matter where you are and what you are doing.

Walking is such an easy and efficient form of exercise, there's no wonder that it's becoming one of the most popular choices of physical activity today. People are beginning to realize that "exercise" doesn't have to be some forced, laborious effort that you drag yourself to the gym to do.

Instead, you can gradually incorporate exercise "movement" into your daily routine and yet receive the same benefits as a 30-minute jaunt on the treadmill. In this chapter, I will help you to see ways to adopt walking (and movement in general) into your day and your life in general.

The Automobile Dilemma

When it comes to physical activity, one of the obstacles Americans face today is our dependency on our cars. We have become very subservient to our four-wheel friends, so much so that we think nothing of driving only two or three blocks to a location. It's "easier" to deal with traffic, tickets, and parking problems than it is to face the thought of walking the three miles to work. Unfortunately, urban developers are encouraging vehicular dependence even more by building cities and towns without sidewalks!

Fortunately, you can make some small changes to help phase out the habit of driving everywhere you go—and that will mean getting more exercise at the same time!

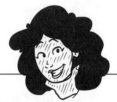

Interesting Excerpts

"Many communities have no sidewalks, and nowhere to walk to, which is bad for public safety as well as for our nation's physical health. It has become impossible in such settings for neighbors to greet one another on the street, or for kids to walk to their own nearby schools. A gallon of gas can be used up just driving to get a gallon of milk. All of these add up to more stress for already-overstressed family lives."

—Vice President Al Gore speaking about the impact of sprawl development on our lives during a speech announcing the Clinton Administration's new Smart Growth proposals on January 11, 1999

Parking Waaaaay Far Away

I work at a gym in Northern California. Like any high-end workout facility, the gym offers a parking garage just beneath the building for its members. It always amazes me to observe how people fight for the parking space closest to the entrance. Despite the fact that they have driven all the way to the gym for the sole purpose of getting some exercise, they struggle to save themselves the effort of having to walk just a few more steps from a parking spot several lanes over. The scary thing is, I don't think that they even realize what they are doing. It has become second nature to take the "path of least resistance" when it comes to physical effort.

If you must drive to your destination, then start changing where you can. Park as far away as you can once you get there so you can get some exercise by walking to and from your car. If you are in a parking lot, choose a space toward the end of the lot. If you park in a parking garage with several floors, drive to the very top so you can walk down and then up the stairs. If you're driving with a friend or in a carpool, have them drop you off several blocks from work and walk the rest of the way. These are little changes that can make a big difference over time, especially when combined with other modifications.

Walking Instead of Driving

If you don't have to drive, don't! Walking to and from work or errands is an excellent way to incorporate exercise into your routine. I've known people who have moved to large cities and had to sell their cars because parking was impossible. After an initial period of adjustment, almost everybody claimed that it was one of the best moves they'd made. In addition to feeling healthier and more energetic, many also claimed to have dropped 5 or 10 pounds without even thinking about it.

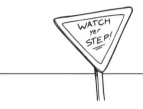

Walkers Watch Out!

Movement of any kind is better than no movement at all. Humankind was built to move. Movement keeps our system in tune, bringing in nutrients and taking out toxins. Without movement, our bodies remain in a state of inertia and stagnancy.

Walking to the grocery store, to work, to meet a friend, or to run errands does take more time, which is what prevents some people from taking advantage of the opportunity. With so much emphasis on time-saving technology, it seems almost archaic to go backward and do things the "old-fashioned" way. Besides, who has the time? But, despite the fact that we are spending so much money trying to "save time," we're busier than we've ever been. Instead of taking advantage of the time we've saved, we end up just filling it up with more things to do.

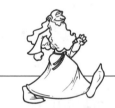

Wise Walkers

With gas prices today, walking to work is not only a healthier option, but a cheaper one, too!

We have to start changing the way we think. We must realize that our sedentary lifestyles are contributing to a number of health problems, so much so that some health professionals consider our lack of movement part of a national epidemic. If you're serious about your health, try to find ways to add movement to your day. Getting rid of your driving habit is one of the best places to start.

Going Up? The Stairs

The gym where I currently work is a large three-story building. When I first started working there, I promised that I would never take the elevator and that, no matter how many times I had to, I'd always take the stairs. For the first year, I stuck to my promise and would, on certain days, have to scale the stairs four or five times an hour. Needless to say, I got into pretty good shape (and even lost a couple of pounds without changing my eating habits).

As much as I hate to admit it, I now find myself, more often than not, pushing that little button and waiting impatiently for the elevator doors to open. Sometimes I will wait five minutes. Five whole minutes! I could be up and down those stairs a number of times in that amount of time, and get a good workout, too. Even personal trainers have their faults!

No matter how fit you are, walking stairs is always going to get your heart rate up. If you typically take the elevator or escalator, try the stairs for a change. Make a commitment to yourself to walk any time it's possible. If you work in a building that is 27 flights high, start by walking the stairs a third of the distance. Increase by a flight every other week. If going down the stairs hurts your knees, it's okay to take the elevator. Just make sure you don't take it on the way up. Rather than calling a co-worker two floors down, walk down to talk to her. If you don't need to use your phone or e-mail, then don't. Walk to that person's desk instead. Take the stairs instead of the elevator or escalator at the airport, mall, hotel, and parking garage.

Digesting Dinner: Taking a Post-Meal Walk

How many times have you pushed yourself back from the dinner table feeling full and tired with only one thing in mind ... TV! When you eat, your blood travels down to your stomach in an attempt to speed up the digestion process. With less blood and oxygen flowing through the rest of your body and brain, you end up feeling tired and sleepy. After sitting at the dinner table, you move a few feet to sit in front of the TV for a couple hours, and then later you slither a few more feet to lie in bed. With so much inactivity, it's no wonder all of that food just seems to sit in your stomach, giving you a bellyache.

Going for a post-meal walk is an excellent way to decrease that full and lethargic feeling. The physical activity increases blood flow, which speeds up the process of digestion while giving you a little boost of energy at the same time. Plus, it's a good way to fit a little exercise in if you've spent the entire day sitting at your desk. Going for a stroll after dinner is a good opportunity to walk the dog, to spend some "play" time with the kids, or to just have a moment to yourself to ponder the day's activities.

Walkers Watch Out!

Imagine when your plumbing stops working. Remember all the trash and waste that builds up? Given enough time, bacteria and strange smells begin to form. Well, without adequate movement, this is what can happen to your body if your bloodstream doesn't recycle enough.

Wise Walkers

To avoid the 4 o'clock slump, try walking up and down several flights of stairs instead of having another cup of coffee or handful of candy. Sugar and caffeine offer the quickest zap of energy to our tiring minds, which is why we crave them for that afternoon snack. A quick jaunt up and down the stairs, however, will increase oxygen flow to your head and literally "feed" your brain, leaving it (and you) feeling more energetic.

Walking to Work

Walking to work is a great way to start the day. In addition to providing you with your daily dose of exercise, it is a good time to sort through the agenda for the day without the distraction of traffic or crowded trains. The problem most people have with walking to work is that it takes too darn long. Having to get up an hour earlier just to walk to work seems crazy, when taking the car will get you there in half the time. Not only will you be able to sleep in, but you won't be all sweaty when you get to work either.

Walking to work definitely has advantages and disadvantages. But, in my humble opinion, the pros far outweigh the cons. For starters, it cuts down on parking and gas costs. Parking can cost several hundred dollars a month, particularly if you're working in "the big city." With gas prices so high these days, filling up the tank is synonymous with emptying out your wallet. Together, these costs add up to quite a bit of money.

And how about safety? Highway driving these days can be hazardous to your health. With so many cars on the road (combined with all of the stress of the people driving them), auto accidents are bound to happen. In fact, they've become a regular part of our early-morning and late-afternoon commute. *Road rage* is a major problem. Angry drivers who use their driving anonymity to commit aggressive acts like cutting you off, flipping you the bird, or suddenly speeding past you just to vent their frustrations have become ordinary occurrences. A lot of the road rage has to do with work stress and an increase in traffic. People are working longer hours, spending more time on the road, and generally having less time to relax and reap the rewards of all their hard labor. It's no wonder we are all feeling a little high-strung.

Perhaps you can see why walking rather than driving to work might be a safer option, if you have the choice to do so. In addition to eliminating your chances of being involved in an auto accident, it also enables you to have some time to "chill out" both before and after work. It gets your blood going and your oxygen flowing, which helps your body rid itself of joint and muscle stiffness

Wise Walkers

You could also try taking a pre-dinner walk. This is a good time, particularly if you're watching what you eat, to separate the day's events from your hunger so that you can sit down and enjoy what you eat and actually taste the food.

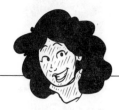

Interesting Excerpts

According to the National Highway Traffic Safety Administration (NHTSA), an estimated 6,289,000 police-reported crashes occurred in 1999, along with an estimated 3,200,000 injured persons the same year.

that comes from sitting at your desk all day. Finally, it saves you a little bit of cash, money with which you can buy a nice pair of walking shoes. If you have the opportunity to walk to work, do. You don't have to jump in with both feet. Start out by walking just one or two days. See how you feel. Give your body a chance to adjust to the change. Add a day every two weeks until you are walking to work every day.

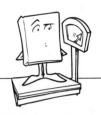

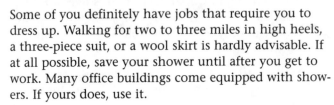

Weighty Words

The phrase **road rage** entered the English language around 1994 in London. The *Oxford English Dictionary* first started listing "road rage" in 1997. It defines it as "a violent anger caused by the stress and frustration of driving in heavy traffic."

Some of you definitely have jobs that require you to dress up. Walking for two to three miles in high heels, a three-piece suit, or a wool skirt is hardly advisable. If at all possible, save your shower until after you get to work. Many office buildings come equipped with showers. If yours does, use it.

If you must walk in your work clothes, that's okay, too. Although not the "fashion statement" of the year, I recommend wearing a good pair of walking shoes to and from the office. Carry your work shoes in your bag. You might need to compromise style for comfort a little and choose clothes that are a little more "suitable" for walking. Try buying fabrics that move with you and that allow your skin to breathe. Remember, this is your health we're talking about. Try to be as flexible as possible. Change may feel strange at first, but you'll get used to it if you're consistent.

Energizing Errands

Everyone has errands. There is always something you "have" to do that you never seem to have time to do. Errands can consist of almost anything from grocery shopping to going to the dry cleaner to making a bank deposit. Yet, how many times have you found yourself stuck in your car waiting for a parking space while running your errands? Or how about parking in the "red zone" to quickly jump in and grab something from the grocery store and coming out to find a ticket waiting for you on your windshield?

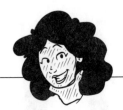

Interesting Excerpts

I have a friend who thought she could get away with parking in a red zone while she jumped out to do a little errand that would only take "a few." She came back to the car to find a cop who had just finished writing her a parking ticket, which cost over $200 and a day's worth of traffic school.

Instead of using up precious time, money, and patience by driving, why don't you try completing your errands on foot? No tickets, no waiting for parking spaces, no traffic; plus, you are taking a step toward better health—all in one. What more could you ask for? Group your errands by location. This way you can do several errands at once and get your walking workout in simultaneously. Talk about saving time!

Pacing It with a Pup

Taking the dog for a walk these days usually means letting him "do his business" on the front lawn, and then turning around and going back inside once he's done. Who has the time and energy to take the dog for a walk, especially after working a 10-hour day? You're tired, grouchy, and just plain "not in the mood." I know. But if you're not going to take Fido out, who will? Just like any living creature, dogs need to exercise, too—especially if they've been cooped up in the house all day long. Plus, it's a good excuse to get you out there, too. And you can skip the dog parks. Although dog parks are great places for your canine to socialize, they aren't designed for walking. The idea is to walk your dog and yourself. Here are some things to remember when promenading with your pup:

1. Bring a leash. Certain areas prohibit dogs from running leash-less. Plus, if you're sticking to city streets, a leash will reduce the risk of your dog getting hit by a car.

2. Carry water, for yourself and for your dog. Use your hands for a cup or bring a small Tupperware bowl.

3. Take a break in the shade if it's hot. Dogs can't sweat and may need a little down-time to cool off.

4. Bring a pooper-scooper to clean up your dog's mess. A plastic bag and gloves will also be helpful.

5. If you are walking trails, check with the local parks first to see whether they allow dogs. Most parks do, but some don't.

I'm not advising you to go out and buy or adopt a dog today. Owning a dog is a big responsibility. In addition to needing exercise, they require food, vet visits, grooming, and attention. If you already have a dog, that's great. But if you are running out the door to buy or adopt one just because you want to ensure your walking habit, I suggest you give it a little more thought. Borrow a neighbor's canine or offer to walk a friend's dog. Get a feel for what it's like to own a dog before rushing out and getting one yourself.

Wise Walkers

In addition to never calling to cancel, canines are good companions because they reduce your risk of being accosted.

Shaping Up While Shopping

What better way to get in shape than to do it while you're shopping? Many mall buildings open up a couple hours earlier than the stores do, so you'll have the place to yourself—and also be the first one in the stores to shop. Certain special clubs and organizations encourage mall walking. Free blood-pressure checks, low-cost or free cholesterol screenings, and presentations by health and exercise experts are just some of the things malls offer to keep you coming back. These clubs are organized individually, so call or visit your local mall to see if they have an organized program for walking. Following are some advantages of walking at the mall:

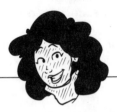

➤ **Out of the weather.** Inside a climate-controlled mall, walkers can dress comfortably and not worry about wind, rain, snow, ice, or heat.

➤ **Away from the traffic.** No intersections to cross, no broken glass or bushes obstructing the path, no auto fumes or rush hour.

➤ **Security.** Walking with others and with mall security on duty.

➤ **Restrooms and water.** Always nearby in the mall.

As you can see, you can incorporate more walking into your life in many ways. Whether you decide to walk to and from work, meander through the mall, climb the stairs instead of taking the elevator, promenade with the pup, or just take an evening stroll after dinner, you will be taking action toward better health as you incorporate more movement into your daily living.

Interesting Excerpts

"Don't stop! An active lifestyle is not something to do for a few days, weeks, or months, and then forget. Make physical activity a lifetime commitment. If you stop exercising, the beneficial effects are rapidly lost. Maintaining good cardiovascular fitness is an ongoing process."

—The American Heart Association

The Least You Need to Know

➤ Park far away to encourage more walking.

➤ Take the stairs instead of the elevator.

➤ Doing errands on foot is a good way to incorporate more movement into your week.

➤ Taking the dog for a walk is a good excuse for you to get some exercise, too!

➤ Getting fit while shopping is fun and good for you.

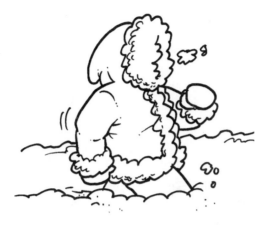

Chapter 18

The Weathered Walker

> ### In This Chapter
>
> ➤ Ways to layer while walking in the cold
>
> ➤ Why hydration is important
>
> ➤ Understanding the difference between heat and humidity
>
> ➤ Wearing clothing that breathes when it's hot
>
> ➤ Ways to make walking in the wet work

Weather should not discourage you from achieving your walking goals, especially since you'll most likely have to contend with fluctuating seasons no matter where you live. Whether you live in the sunny West, the snowy East, the humid South, or the rainy Northwest, you can find ways to work around the weather to maintain your exercise regimen.

Wearing clothes that protect you from the sun, snow, wind, and rain, as well as learning where and what time to work out, are important things to know ahead of time. Staying well-hydrated and wearing clothes that "breathe" are other details to remember, no matter what kind of weather. In this chapter, I'll guide you through three environmental conditions (cold, heat, and rain) and show you how you can take better care of the inside, as well as the outside, of your body in order to continue your walking routine safe and sound all year 'round.

A Winter Walking Wonderland

Cold weather does not automatically mean you have a good excuse not to walk. In fact, walking in the winter can be quite inspiring. White-covered mountains, silent forests, and the bright sunlight reflecting off the snow are beautiful sights to see during your winter walks. The cold, crisp air is often energizing and invigorating, making you feel alive and exhilarated. Plus, it's a good excuse to get out of the house and avoid that "cooped-up" feeling so commonly associated with winter.

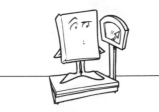

Weighty Words

Hypothermia means heat loss or low body temperature.

But if you're going to walk in the winter, you must consider a few things first. *Hypothermia* is a big concern for winter walkers. When the environment in which you walk is cold, you must protect your body from losing too much heat. First, you can layer your clothing to keep your body insulated, and you'll need to stay hydrated because, yes, you do sweat in the cold, too!

Clothing for the Cold

The most important factor for walkers to consider when getting dressed for their winter walks is layering. Layering offers you the luxury of staying warm when it's cold out and peeling off as you warm up. But just wrapping yourself up in "any old thing" you happen to find around the house is not a good idea. There is an art to layering so that your clothing will absorb and "wick" moisture away from your body, keep you warm, and allow your skin to breathe, while protecting you from the elements. This "art" of layering is described in Chapter 4, "Gathering Your Gear." Please refer to it for suggestions on how to layer wisely.

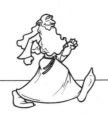

Wise Walkers

You might consider taking a backpack along with you. This will enable you to carry extra clothing, accessories, water, and an umbrella without tying up your hands.

If you are accustomed to wearing pants, consider slipping on an extra layer first. A pair of tights or long underwear will provide additional warmth. Try to wear loose pants so you can move around easily. You might also contemplate wearing a turtleneck to protect your neck from the cold. Again, choose a fabric that absorbs sweat and dries quickly. Wear a short-sleeve shirt underneath so you can take the turtleneck off if it gets too hot.

Keeping your hands, feet, and head warm is also very important. Colder temperatures cause blood to be directed away from the hands and feet to the center of the body to keep the internal organs warm and protected. This is why your hands and feet feel so cold when walking in chillier conditions. The following are some suggestions for winter-wear accessories:

➤ Hats keep the heat in and protect the head from rain and snow.

➤ Gloves warm your hands and help protect your fingers from freezing.

➤ Ear bands or muffs protect the ears from cold wind, snow, and rain.

➤ Scarves keep your neck and upper chest warm.

➤ An umbrella holds back rain, hail, or snow.

➤ Lip balm and sunscreen protect you from the sun and wind.

It is important that in addition to being warm, you're also comfortable. Clothing that restricts movement, causes profuse perspiration, or holds in moisture, is probably going to make your walking experience miserable. Before going out and buying a whole new wardrobe (some of these fabrics can be quite costly), try a few different types first. Choose the ones you like and feel most comfy in, and go from there.

Hydration

Many people make the mistake of not drinking enough water during their winter walks; there's something about the cold that tricks them into thinking that they don't need to. But you do sweat when you are exercising, be it hot or cold, and you do need to replace those lost fluids in order to stay healthy. If you don't, you run the risk of becoming *dehydrated,* a condition that can sometimes be hard to detect. In fact, by the time you feel "thirsty," you're already dehydrated. So make sure you hydrate adequately before, during, and after each of your walks.

To avoid becoming dehydrated, you must be proactive and drink plenty of water ahead of time, not just when you're thirsty. A good habit is to drink a glass of water every hour throughout the day and about 10 minutes before each walk. You will also want to carry a water bottle with you so that you'll have liquid on hand. Drink at least 5 to 8 ounces every 15 to 20 minutes. Here are some suggestions for carrying water with you:

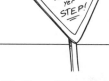

Walkers Watch Out!

Some of the more common signs of dehydration include nausea after exercise; dark yellow or no urine; a dry, sticky mouth; and/or dry eyes.

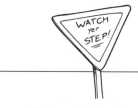

Walkers Watch Out!

Avoid beverages that have caffeine. Coffee, cocoa, cola, and some teas are diuretics and cause you to lose fluids.

➤ Buy a hip/waist pack that has an external bottle holder attached to it.

➤ Carry a backpack for storing your water bottle.

➤ A platypus water holder is a plastic container that flattens when empty and rounds when it is full.

➤ A camelback is a container that you carry on your back, and has a plastic tube you keep in (or near) your mouth that provides a steady stream of liquid.

➤ If you are using a refillable water bottle, make sure you clean it with warm water and soap after every use to prevent the spread of germs.

Know the Snow: Ice vs. Powder

There is nothing more beautiful than walking through a snow-covered forest. The silence and peace of the fresh morning snow brings a sense of tranquility unlike anything else. But snow turns into ice and ice can be dangerously slippery (not to mention hard), and falling can cause injury that is both painful and disabling.

Wise Walkers

Using a pair of ski poles while walking in the snow offers balance as well as providing a good walking aid through especially deep snow.

If you live in an area where snow is common, you might want to invest in some specialty shoes that have good traction to stop you quickly on snow and ice. You might consider going as far as purchasing a pair of crampons or snow shoes if you live in an especially snowy area. In addition to proper shoes, good sunglasses and sunscreen are two other important accessories to take along. The white snow may be beautiful, but its brightness can also cause blindness and severe sunburn if you aren't careful.

Heated Hikes

I have the advantage of living in a pretty moderate climate here in Northern California. It never really gets too hot (or too cold, for that matter) to exercise. But many of you live in the southern states and in the middle of the county, with summer heat conditions: temperatures that soar well into the 90s and above. Most people opt not to exercise in these conditions for fear of heat illness, not to mention the fact that it's just plain uncomfortable. So, you put off your program for a couple of months hoping that you will find the motivation to start again come autumn.

What happens to your body in the heat, and why is it so darn hard to exercise? Basically, as the heat rises outside your body, the temperature inside rises as well. In an attempt to maintain "normal" body temperature, your blood will release water and heat (perspiration), which helps to keep the skin cool and your body temperature down through evaporation. With less water in your blood, your blood volume decreases, which forces the heart to work harder (beat faster) in order to deliver adequate oxygen and blood to the working muscles. The following is a list of some of the illnesses associated with heat stress:

➤ **Heat cramps.** Painful contractions of the muscles, usually in the abdomen and the legs.

➤ **Heat exhaustion.** Caused from the loss of fluids and sodium due to excessive heat. Symptoms include heavy perspiration, vomiting, pale and clammy skin, weakness, and fainting.

➤ **Heat syncope.** Fainting or weakness due to excessive heat.

➤ **Heat stroke.** Heat strokes usually occur after heat exhaustion; the body is unable to lose heat, so the body temp rises above 106°F. Symptoms include: rapid heart beat; red, hot, dry skin; confusion; and loss of consciousness.

Although the conditions mentioned above should be considered serious, they do not mean that you must completely stop exercising until cooler conditions arrive. There are tricks and ways to work around the heat that will enable you to continue your program safely. We will discuss these later in this chapter.

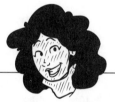

Interesting Excerpts

When you work out, your muscles' demand for blood increases, which also forces the heart to work harder. When you work out during hot conditions, your heart is working twice as hard to deliver blood to the harder-working muscles as well as blood (and water) to the capillaries under the skin's surface in an attempt to keep the body cool. This is why your heart rate increases so substantially in hotter weather. If you throw dehydration into the equation, you could potentially have a very dangerous situation on your hands.

Heat Index and Humidity

Humidity is another concern for walkers. Humidity will hinder the evaporation of perspiration. Remember that perspiration releases heat from our bodies through evaporation. As relative humidity rises, the evaporation (cooling) rate decreases, putting you

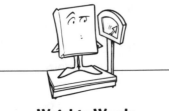

Weighty Words

Humidity refers to the amount of moisture in the air. The more vapor, the less evaporation of perspiration.

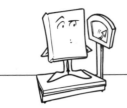

Weighty Words

Water weight refers to the number of pounds gained or lost by water retention and/or evaporation.

at risk for heat illnesses like those mentioned earlier. Choose times of the day when the temperature and humidity tend to be lower.

Hydration: Staying Cool Inside

One of the best ways to protect your body from heat illness is to stay hydrated—drink lots of water. The evaporation of perspiration keeps you cool, but you must have water in your system in order to sweat. Make sure to drink fluids—and in particular water—before, during, and after your walk. In addition, drink 16 ounces of water for every pound of *water weight* lost during activity. Drink an extra eight ounces for every caffeinated beverage you consume per day. If you plan to walk for several hours at a time, bring a sports drink along with your regular dose of water. Exercising for prolonged periods of time decreases levels of sodium and sugar in your bloodstream, which can cause not only a drop in energy but in blood pressure as well.

Keep a bottle of water with you at all times. Make sure it is enough to last you the entire workout. Cold water is better, because it will help cool you down. You might want to consider putting a bottle of water in the freezer the night before your walk. Make sure you take it out a couple hours beforehand so you'll have some liquid to sip from.

Ventilation: Clothing That Breathes

Carrying water with you is your number-one priority when walking in the heat. But you can do other things to protect your body from excessive heat as well. What you wear makes a big difference in defending yourself against excessive heat. You must choose clothes that allow your body not only to breathe but also to transfer moisture from your skin's surface to the environment. Fabrics that "wick" sweat away, such as CoolMax and Supplex, are good items to start with. You might also consider buying lighter-colored clothing since they tend to reflect, rather than absorb, heat. Finally, wear clothing that is looser-fitting, to increase airflow and reduce heat. Light, loose-fitting long-sleeve shirts are a good idea because they protect your skin from sunburn and heat. (For more information about fabrics suitable for walking, see Chapter 4.)

Wise Walkers

Drink fluids before, during, and after your walk. About a pint (16 fluid ounces) before exercise, and about 1 cup every 15 minutes during aerobic exercise. If you walk for over an hour, you might want to consider taking a sports drink that has some carbohydrates in it, such as Gatorade. This way you will have a little pick-me-up when you're feeling sluggish. You can make your own sports drink by dissolving a tablespoon of sugar and a pinch of salt in a tablespoon of orange juice or in two tablespoons of lemon juice, then adding 7$\frac{1}{2}$ ounces of cold water and stiring.

Protecting Your Head: Hats and Other Accessories

In addition to wearing light and loose clothing, you can also investigate the possibility of accessorizing your walking outfit to defend against the heat and sun. Hats are an excellent way to keep the sun out of your eyes and the heat off your head and face. Choose a hat that's big enough to give your head enough room to "breathe" and perspire. A tight-fitting hat may trap heat in as well as give you a headache. Try to find one that has a sweatband sewn into it to prevent sweat from dripping into your eyes.

Sunglasses and sunscreen are also very important "accessories" to remember when the "heat is on." Always lather up with sunscreen before going out in the sun. Take a bottle with you just in case. Watch out for lotions that clog your pores and don't allow your skin to perspire. If you sweat profusely, make sure you reapply, since you are likely to wipe a lot of the sunscreen off while dabbing the sweat away. You might as well throw some sunglasses on while applying the sunscreen. Shades that protect your eyes from UVA and UVB rays may reduce the chance of developing cataracts later in life. Plus, squinting for an hour or more from bright sunlight is hardly very comfortable.

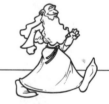

Wise Walkers

Some hats come with flaps sewn down the back to protect your neck from the sun. If you walk in unprotected, open spaces, you might want to consider purchasing one of these to protect your neck from sunburn.

You can reduce your risk of sunburn and sunstroke by timing your walk well. There is hot and then there is HOT. And the "hottest" time of day usually falls between 10 A.M. and 3 P.M., especially at noon when the sun is at its highest point. If you have no choice but to walk outdoors during the warmer months, then choose times during the day when the sun is not so strong. Usually before 10 A.M. and after 4 P.M. are best.

Damp Tramps

Walking in the rain is not as crazy as it sounds. Most people stop dead in their tracks at any sight of rain and will not even attempt exercising outdoors until it has stopped. But walking in the rain can be done, and it can be done comfortably and dryly if you are dressed properly. Besides, rain is just water, and a little water never hurt anyone, right?

Appropriate Attire

Wearing the right gear is the most important factor to consider before walking in the rain. Staying dry is crucial for comfort, so you must choose clothing that keeps the warmth in and the wet out. Cotton, for example, is not a good material to wear in the rain since it absorbs moisture so easily and doesn't dry quickly. Outer rainwear must be waterproof. Wearing a jacket or poncho large enough to cover the majority of your upper body, including your neck and head, is a good idea. You can find plastic ponchos that fold up into small envelopes at most sports or thrift stores for less than five dollars.

Another option you have is a waterproof-treated jacket. Most of these jackets are made of nylon or polyester on the outside and have a thin waterproof lining on the inside. The following are some things to look for when shopping for a raincoat:

1. Vents and air holes under arms to allow "breathing"
2. Hood and neck protection (collar)
3. A drawstring around the waist to adjust fit
4. Waterproof pockets with a zipper and a flap
5. Factory-sealed seams

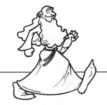

Wise Walkers

Another interesting accessory you might think about purchasing is the Arctic Bandana. This nifty little gadget is a tube of fabric filled with a special water-absorbing gel that expands to many times its size. When you wear it around your neck or head, it cools you by evaporation. You can order by calling, toll-free, 1–888–767–SGMC (7462).

Walkers Watch Out!

Rain means lower visibility, especially for drivers. Wear brighter colors and/or reflective clothing, and pay extra attention when crossing the street.

The same rules that apply for upper-body gear goes for lower-body wear. Vinyl pants that zip up the side are sold for a reasonable price at most sporting goods stores. Because vinyl is not a "breathable" fabric, you will not want to wear it on long, fast-paced walks where you sweat a lot. Make sure you slip a pair of moisture-"wicking" tights underneath them to minimize the amount of moisture on your skin. Other laminated, waterproof fabrics like Gore-Tex and Sympatex, which can be relatively expensive, are great because they allow your skin to breathe while wicking moisture away. Whatever material you choose, make sure that the pants fit comfortably. A tight pair of pants will restrict movement and can be very uncomfortable.

Keeping your head dry (and warm) is smart, especially if you are thinking about spending an extended amount of time walking in the rain. You can do several things to protect your head:

➤ Wear hats that are made of waterproof material like Gore-Tex or other laminated fabric.

➤ Buy a hooded jacket.

➤ Spray your favorite hat with a waterproof treatment like Scotchgard.

➤ Use plastic rain-hoods that don't obstruct your vision.

➤ Buy a small portable umbrella that can withstand some wind.

Covering Your Feet

Almost as important as protecting your head is protecting your feet. Walking in shoes that are soaked through with rain can cause much discomfort, chafing, and sometimes blisters. You can do several things to prevent your feet from getting (and staying) wet. First, you can buy shoes that are waterproof. Gore-Tex–lined shoes and boots keep the wet out while allowing your feet to breathe. You can also seal your own walking shoes with a waterproof treatment like Sno-Seal (for leather) or Scotchgard and Tectron for nylon. Although not as fool-proof as the Sno-Seal, these "home treatments" work better than nothing to slow the rain from soaking inside the shoe.

In addition to keeping the outside of your shoes dry, you can prevent foot soakage by wearing protective socks. There is nothing worse than wearing a pair of socks that, after becoming saturated with water, swell up and cause chafing and blisters. To prevent such tragedies from occurring, you can do a number of things. You can purchase socks made

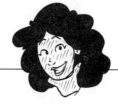

Interesting Excerpts

Did you know that cotton fiber retains three times the moisture of acrylic and 14 times the moisture of CoolMax? In descending order of moisture-absorption ranking, the following fibers are listed: cotton, wool, acrylic, CoolMax, polypropylene.

of wicking materials, such as polypropylene and acrylic, that pull moisture away from the foot. CoolMax, SmartWool, and Thorlo are good brands to look for moisture control, warmth, and comfort. You might consider buying a pair of waterproof socks as well. SealSkinz makes a waterproof sock that keeps the wet out if you decide not to waterproof your shoes.

The Least You Need to Know

➤ Use three basic layers of clothing for cold-weather walking.

➤ Cotton absorbs and holds on to moisture.

➤ High relative humidity can make it feel hotter than it actually is.

➤ Clothes that allow your skin to breathe are important for warm-weather walks.

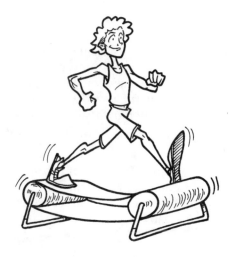

Exercising Your Alternatives

Given the choice, most people would opt to walk outdoors rather than exercise inside. The beauty of nature, fresh air, and a change of scenery are all good reasons to walk in the wilderness. But not everyone chooses, nor has the ability, to share wonder in the wild. Weather conditions, time of day, lack of access to natural parks, and just a general preference for being at home are some of the reasons why people choose to exercise indoors. Whatever your reasons, staying inside does not have to hinder your exercise and walking plans.

With just a few tools and a lot of imagination, you can create a walking and workout program for yourself regardless of whether you are at home or at the gym. Knowing what resources you have and how to access them, as well as keeping an open mind, will result in a safe, effective, and fun workout comparable to any outdoor activity. In this chapter, we will explore some of those resources.

Home Is Where the Heart Is

Having the home alternative for exercise is good insurance. Since exercise is to become a lifetime activity, chances are you will not be able to make it outside or to the gym for your ritual walk now and then. Perhaps you have to stay home with Junior to take care of his cold or wait for the deliveryman to bring the new dryer. You want to exercise to keep your body movin' and your exercise habit groovin', but you don't have the option to leave the house.

One does not have to belong to a gym or become an outdoors enthusiast in order to get in shape. The home is a great arena for fitness. All you really need is a treadmill and you're ready to go.

Treadmills are convenient and consistent. In addition to being accessible, they are easy to control. The terrain, incline, and speed all remain the same unless you change them. You also can see exactly how fast and far you walk and how many calories you burn with each minute, features that walking outdoors does not offer. Lastly, you can entertain yourself with TV, a good book, or a magazine while walking on the treadmill. You can talk on the phone, wait for the delivery man, or keep an eye on the kids, too.

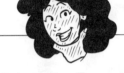

Interesting Excerpts

Treadmills are the most popular means of home exercise equipment today, capturing 33 percent of home fitness equipment sales, according to *Sporting Goods Business Magazine*.

Walkers Watch Out!

Do not exchange safety for entertainment. I have seen people get very carried away with conversations, music, and even while reading a book while walking on the treadmill. If your foot catches a place off the moving belt, and you're not paying attention, you could cause some serious damage. Pay attention to where you are walking at all times.

Terrific Treadmill Treds

Simple, easy to operate, and an excellent way to burn calories, treadmills have not lost their popularity despite the many new and trendy machines being introduced to the fitness industry today. You have no limit to the different kinds of workouts you can perform on treadmills. From flat, slow strolls to hilly hikes, treadmills offer a wide variety of challenges for novice and seasoned walkers alike. Let's take a look at some walking workouts while on the treadmill.

A Beginner's Base

If you are brand new to the treadmill, you will want to start off flat; don't worry about the inclines until after you've gotten used to walking on a moving surface. The most important thing to remember for the beginner is to stay balanced and to keep your feet on the belt. Start off at 1 mile per hour and gradually increase the speed. Remember that the treadmill sometimes takes time to catch up. If you increase the speed, do it slowly. Wait until the treadmill (and you) are stabilized at the new pace before you turn it up a notch again.

Try to walk as naturally as possible. At first, you might want to use the handrails for support, but don't get used to relying on them too much. The idea is to walk as naturally as possible. You will notice that it seems a little awkward in the beginning, especially at the slower paces. Just try to relax and let your feet fall naturally. The following are guidelines for maintaining proper form while walking on a treadmill:

➤ Your focus should be straight ahead with your head centered between your shoulders.

➤ Keep your back straight, your chest lifted, and your shoulders square.

➤ Keep your belly taut by gently pulling your stomach in toward your spine. Make sure that you are not pushing out by holding your breath.

➤ Your arms should be bent close to 90 degrees and should remain close to your body. Your forearm in front of you should come parallel with the floor. Your back upper arm should swing far enough back so that your fist is in line with your hips.

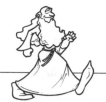

Wise Walkers

When you start the treadmill, make sure you are not standing on the belt. Place your feet on either side of the belt, so that when you start it up you won't be knocked off balance by the movement of the ground beneath you.

Beginners should walk no more than 20 to 30 minutes at a time on the treadmill. Starting out with two or three days a week is probably a good idea. Other than balance and coordination, try concentrating on building a base at a moderate speed (2.5 to 3.0 mph) with no incline. After three to four weeks, you can start playing with the speed, adding a little at a time until you've reached a pace that is challenging but manageable. I suggest adding speed through intervals so that you can allow your body to adjust to the increase slowly. Here is a sample workout:

Beginner's Speed Intervals: 30 Minutes

Phase	Speed	Time
Warm up	2.5 mph	5 minutes
Warm up	2.8 mph	5 minutes
Interval 1	3.0 mph	1 minute

continues

Beginner's Speed Intervals: 30 Minutes (continued)

Phase	Speed	Time
Rest	2.5 mph	1 minute
Rest	2.5 mph	1 minute
Interval 3	3.2 mph	1 minute
Rest	2.5 mph	1 minute
Interval 4	3.2 mph	2 minutes
Rest	2.5 mph	1 minute
Interval 5	3.5 mph	1 minute
Rest	2.5 mph	1 minute
Interval 6	3.5 mph	2 minutes
Rest	2.5 mph	1 minute
Cool down	2.8 mph	2 minutes
Cool down	2.5 mph	3 minutes

Again, you can make this workout longer (and harder) by adding a minute or two to each interval or by adding a couple more intervals, or you can do both. If you are just starting out, remember to progress slowly and not to add too much time too soon.

Something worth mentioning is speed and stride length. Obviously, people with longer legs are going to experience the 3.5 mph differently than those with shorter legs. If you feel that the speed I recommended in the preceding example is too fast or too slow, go ahead and adjust it.

Walkers Watch Out!

Some first-time treadmill users may feel dizzy after getting off the treadmill. This is often due to looking down at the moving belt while walking. If you can, keep your focus ahead. Hold on to the railings if needed, but keep your head up.

Intermediate Inclines

Those of you who have been treading for some time and need a little change to your routine might consider adding inclines. Walking hills works your calves, hamstrings, and buttock muscles more than walking on a flat surface. Plus, walking up an incline is an excellent way to up the ante without having to increase the speed. After all, you can only walk so fast before you have to start jogging. If you want to vary your routine, work different muscles in your legs, or have reached your "speed limit," then adding inclines to your weekly walks is a good idea. The following is a sample 30-minute incline workout. If you want to walk longer, or increase the intensity of your workout, you can either add the number of intervals or lengthen the time of each interval.

Intermediate Incline Workout

Phase	Speed	Incline	Time
Warm up	3.0 mph	0.0%	5 minutes
Warm up	3.5 mph	2.0%	5 minutes
Interval	3.5 mph	4.0%	2 minutes
Rest	3.5 mph	0.0%	1 minute
Interval 2	3.5 mph	4.0%	2 minutes
Rest	3.5 mph	0.0%	1 minute
Interval 3	3.5 mph	6.0%	2 minutes
Rest	3.5 mph	0.0%	2 minutes
Interval 4	3.5 mph	6.0%	2 minutes
Rest	3.5 mph	0.0%	2 minutes
Interval 5	3.5 mph	8.0%	1 minute
Rest	3.5 mph	4.0%	2 minutes
Cool down	3.0 mph	0.0%	3 minutes

If you are new to inclines, start out by adding 1 or 2 percent grade at a time. After a 5- to 10-minute warm up at no grade at all, increase the pace so that it is comfortable but challenging, somewhere between 2.5 and 3.5 mph. Add 2 percent after you've warmed up. Continue to add 1 or 2 percent every 1 or 2 minutes. Don't exceed a 3 or 4 percent grade for your first several tries. Stay at the same pace the entire time. Do not adjust your speed. Let your body get used to the grade first. Whether you are aware of it or not, the slight incline does put added stress on your lower back, so you'll want to be careful of the rate at which you progress.

Advanced Adventures

To turn an intermediate workout into an advanced one, you can do one of several things. You can add speed and incline simultaneously rather than alternating between the two. In other words, you can continue to add increments of speed and grade until you are walking as fast and as steep as you can manage. Walking at 4.0 mph on a 6 percent grade is going to get your heart rate up and give your legs a good work-over, believe me. The longer the intervals, the harder it will be. Of course, maintaining high levels of speed and grade is also quite a challenge.

Walkers Watch Out!

Just as with hill walks outdoors, you do not want to do incline walks on the treadmill every time you walk. Vary your program between pace days, flat days, slow days, and incline days.

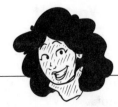

Interesting Excerpts

Another way to increase the challenge of your treadmill workout is to increase the amount of weight you carry on your body. Remember, it takes more energy to carry heavier loads. You can augment your weight by carrying a backpack filled with weights, or you can purchase a weighted vest. A weighted vest is a specially-designed nylon vest that has pockets sewn into it where small two- to five-pound weights are placed. The weights are easy to add and remove so the vest is efficiently adjustable.

In order to safely add speed and hills at the same time, I suggest you do the following: After a 5- to 10-minute warm up at a low grade and a moderate pace (3.0 mph/ 2 percent grade) alternate between adding speed and incline every third minute. Give yourself a minute between each shift to allow your body to adjust to the change. Keep doing this until you reach your desired pace and incline. Generally speaking, a speed between 3.5 and 4.5 mph combined with an incline of 5.0 to 8.0 is a good goal to work toward.

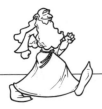

Wise Walkers

Because walking on inclines stretches your Achilles tendons more than walking on flat surfaces, make sure you spend an extra five minutes stretching your calves after each hill walk.

You can also walk with weights to make your treadmill workout more challenging. Hand weights will increase the amount of work your upper body performs. Plus, it forces you to maintain good muscle balance and control, since the weights have a tendency to knock your equilibrium off at first. Finally, carrying weights means that your body will be carrying more mass and burning more calories with each step.

If you decide to carry weights while walking on the treadmill, you must start light. Carrying 15-pound weights while walking fast up an incline is dangerous and could knock you off the treadmill entirely. In addition, if the weights are too heavy, you could do some major muscle damage to your shoulders, neck, and back. Start with a half-pound to one pound at first. It may feel light initially, but after 20 minutes you might be thankful you didn't grab the 5-pounders.

Safety

Treadmills are moving machines. Although you aren't actually going anywhere, your feet sure are moving fast, so you must take certain steps to avoid injury. The following are some tips and some safety precautions you will want to consider before climbing on board a treadmill:

➤ First and foremost, make sure the treadmill has standard safety features, including an emergency shut-off that is easily accessible, the ability to limit incline and speed, a gradual start and stop, and accessible handrails.

➤ See that it has a safe starting speed of .5 mph or less.

➤ In terms of form, let your foot go through its natural "heel to toe" motion. As it contacts the belt, avoid walking flat-footed.

➤ Look straight ahead of you and not down at the belt.

➤ Straddle, rather than stand, on the belt when you are starting up the treadmill.

➤ Don't rely too heavily on the handrails. They are okay to establish balance as you start out but should be abandoned within several minutes after you've begun.

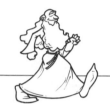

Wise Walkers

You could also purchase a pair of wrist weights if you don't want to carry dumbbells in your hands. Many sporting goods stores sell Velcro wrist weights that attach easily around your wrist, and they range in weight from $1/2$ to 10 pounds.

Keeping Yourself Occupied: Music, Books, and Socializing

One of the biggest complaints that people have about stationary equipment is that they get bored easily. The combination of stagnant scenery and stale air can be a recipe for the doldrums, for sure. So, how can you make your treadmill trek a little more interesting? Now that you've learned the rules and regulations, the ins and the outs of becoming a "true" treadmiller, here are some suggestions on ways to make your stationary workout more entertaining:

➤ Music can be an amazing motivator for some. There's nothing like blasting your favorite tunes while walking in time with the beat. Choose music with a tempo that matches your pace. Music that is too fast or slow might disturb your rhythm. Many gyms have built-in musical stations you can plug into, or you can bring your own music. Just make sure that you don't forget the headphones.

➤ Watching television is another option for those of you who need something to do on the treadmill. Most gyms have one or two TV wall units to share amongst a group of exercisers. Some clubs, however, have taken it to the next level by installing a mini TV monitor at individual exercise station so that people don't have to argue over what shows to watch.

➤ Reading on the treadmill is not recommended since it means that you are looking down rather than forward as advised. Plus, reading means that you are probably holding on to the handrails to stabilize your focus. But despite these warnings, many people choose to read on the treadmill. If you are an avid reader and cannot go anywhere without your book or your magazines, try to read only when walking at slow, lower-intensity levels.

➤ You always have the option of talking with a friend while exercising. A great way to catch up and exercise simultaneously, social sashaying kills two birds with one stone. Make sure you don't get so caught up in the jabber that you lose your concentration or your footing.

➤ Finally, some clubs have become hip to the Internet craze and have attached computer monitors to their exercise equipment where one can, among other things, check e-mail or surf the Web. The same safety warnings apply here as with reading.

Buying a Treadmill

So, you have decided that walking is your thing. You like it and you want to pursue it to the best of your abilities—indoors. Whether you are hibernating from the cold outdoors, hiding from the humid heat, or you just prefer to work out in the privacy of your own home, buying a treadmill is probably a good idea. It's a popular idea, too. According to the U.S. National Sporting Goods Association (NSGA), retail sales of treadmills topped $757 million last year, up from $42 million in 1983. In fact, treadmill exercise is the fastest-growing activity in the country—having increased by 37 percent between 1992 and 1993, and by 348 percent since 1987 (according to Harvey Lauer, president of the research firm of American Sports Data in Hartsdale, New York).

If you are ready to buy a treadmill for your home, you should consider a number of things before you dish out too much (or too little) money:

➤ Be choosy about where you purchase your treadmill. Buy it from a specialty fitness store if possible, rather than from a department store. The salespeople at these specialty sports stores are likely to be more educated about their equipment and should be able to answer most of your questions about your treadmill.

➤ Watch out for misleading terms such as "treadmill duty" and *peak horsepower,* which are usually gimmicks to unrealistically raise the horsepower.

➤ Invest in a good motor. A good motor uses a circuitry that senses belt load, and it communicates with the motor to make necessary adjustments to ensure smooth operation. Pay attention to the smoothness and constancy of the belt as you walk. A simple test you can do is to set the treadmill at a low speed, grasp a railing, and give the belt a little resistance with your foot as though trying to slow the belt. A weak motor will kick up a fuss, indicating that it won't be a smooth operator nor last very long under use. The belt and motor should provide a smooth and continuous motion without jerks or sudden spurts.

➤ Notice the starting speed. A safe starting speed should be .5 mph or less. A starting speed of one mile per hour or more is often too fast for most users and may result in a sudden jerk when the belt is started.

➤ Buy a treadmill with a wide-enough belt. Your average good-sized belt will be around 17 by 48 inches. The thickness of the running belt is important, too. Two-ply belts are stronger and less likely to curl at the sides than are one-ply belts.

➤ Make sure the deck (the length of the running surface) is long enough to allow flexibility in stride length. Longer decks provide room for a more comfortable stride than shorter surfaces.

➤ The treadmill should have good resilience. Resilience is the absorption by the treadmill of the force from the impact of your feet, which helps to relieve the stress on your knees and ankles.

➤ Your treadmill should have a computerized control panel—and the simpler the better. The control panel should be easy to read, with buttons that have simple commands and readouts that are large and easy to find. Electronic feedback displays of speed, time, and distance are generally standard on most treadmills. Some also display the number of calories burned or the heart rate. Also, most treadmills offer preset and/or customizable programming capabilities.

➤ Your treadmill should have an incline feature. Quality incline should be quiet and shouldn't cause the treadmill to wobble at high elevations. Electric incline with rack and pinion is ideal, but a manual crank is more cost effective. Most quality treadmills will incline to 10 percent. Commercial-grade treadmills often go as high as 25 percent, although too high an incline may easily lead to injury. Most users don't go above 10 percent.

➤ Quality treadmills should have a lifetime warranty on the frame, but look for one that also guarantees two or more years on moving

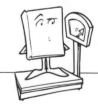

Weighty Words

Peak horsepower is the motor's maximum potential at various moments in usage, but cannot be maintained for a considerable length of time.

parts, especially the belt and rollers, and two or more years on the motor and electronic components as well.

➤ Price: Plan to spend from around $1,000 and up for a quality motorized tread-mill. Below this price range, treadmills do not meet most of the recommended guidelines. You may have also noticed that high-end treadmills average around $3,000 and up, but the competitiveness of the market has produced some excellent treadmills at around $2,000.

The Least You Need to Know

➤ Treadmills are a good substitute for walking outside when the great outdoors is not an option.

➤ A good way to challenge your workout on a treadmill is to combine incline and speed together.

➤ A treadmill should have a starting speed of no more than .5 mph.

➤ You get what you pay for when buying a treadmill.

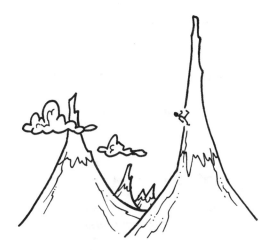

Taking It to the Next Level

Walking is not just an exercise; it's a lifestyle. I've already discussed how incorporating the habit of walking into your life will enhance your health and well-being. Now I'd like to show you how walking can broaden your horizons by introducing you to new cultures, landscapes, and challenges you may never have imagined. Hiking, backpacking, walking vacations, and competitive events are all ways that you can enhance your experience as a walker and as an individual in general. More and more people are realizing how they can incorporate walking into other areas of their lives. Because walking is cheap, easy, and can be done anywhere and anytime, a great number of people are using it as a tool to learn about nature, broaden their scope of the world, or just challenge their own limits.

Take a Walk on the Wild Side

John Muir, the nineteenth-century naturalist, said this of the power of Mother Nature: "Climb the mountains and get their good tidings. Nature's peace will flow into you as sunshine flows into trees. The winds will blow their own freshness into you, and the storms their energy, while cares will drop off like autumn leaves."

Getting away, out from under blaring fluorescent lights and towering skyscrapers, has a way of reviving the spirit. One has a tendency to get so caught up in the hustle and bustle of the city that they forget about the vastness of the land on which they stand.

Hiking and backpacking are great ways to explore the great outdoors, to take a break from traffic and work and to get in touch with nature. They are also great ways to get in and stay in shape. But deciding to venture out for a week, or for even a day trip, takes organization, skill, and preparation. Read on for some tips on how to get the most out of the wonderful world of walking in the wild.

Where to Go? Ideas for Trails and Treks

I did not realize what I was getting myself into as I gleefully typed the word "hiking" in my little search box. The amount of information on backpacking, hiking, trail trekking, and just plain ol' walking in the woods is mind-boggling! Apparently, it's a popular hobby for many people.

You can find cyber information and publications a-plenty, depending on your skill level, how many miles you want to hike, where you want to hike, and what "type" of trail you'd like to traverse. You will find online resources, books, and magazines, as well as state, regional, and national sources, offering you an abundance of information to plan your trip. In addition to this, you will discover that the majority of back-country shops carry maps and information about great places to walk in the area. Most local people feel proud of their natural attractions and are very friendly and happy to discuss their knowledge of their homeland.

Comfortable Clothing and Durable Footwear: To Boot or Not To Boot?

With the exception of shoe type, wilderness wear is essentially the same as other out-door wear. If you're walking in the cold, you must layer. Refer to Chapter 18, "The Weathered Walker," for tips on layering in the cold. If you're walking in the heat, you must cover up and shield yourself from the sun with hats, sunscreen, and long sleeves. If it's going to be wet, make sure you wear something to keep you protected from the rain and snow.

As with any outdoor walking, you must prepare for long walks by bringing an extra change of clothing. Be aware of the type of area you'll be walking in. For example, if the trail is not cut clearly, then you will want to wear long pants to avoid scratches and cuts from overgrown shrub. If you'll be crossing rivers or streams, you might want to bring a pair of shorts or loose pants that can be rolled up. Also, be aware of bugs and other biting creatures, and dress accordingly to protect yourself from being attacked.

In terms of hiking boots, it's probably a good idea to invest in a pair if you're going to be spending a lot of time hiking and backpacking. But what type of boot should you buy? There are several types of boots out there for different levels of hikers. Here are some tips to help you choose the right boot:

➤ Outdoor cross-trainers are for terrain that is fairly more even, and are good for light trail hiking. They are more flexible than regular hiking boots and are often made of the same material as running shoes but in darker materials.

➤ Lightweight hikers are made for hikes up to four hours in duration, and can support backpacks up to 15 pounds. They are more flexible than regular hikers and are commonly made with canvas and leather.

➤ Heavyweight hiking boots are typically made for the more serious backpacker who spends hours, days, and sometimes weeks out in the wild. They are typically made of all leather and are stiffer and more durable than the other two types of boots. Many are waterproof as well.

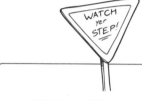

Walkers Watch Out!

Safety is the main concern with hiking boots. Those on sale aren't necessarily the best ones to buy. Expect to pay a fair amount for a decent hiking boot.

Training Tips: Preparing Your Heart for Hiking

Probably the best way to train for hiking and backpacking is to simply get out there and hike and backpack! Research the recreational parks in your area. Find out about the different trails and their difficulty levels. Begin with smaller, shorter hikes and work your way up. And, yes, bring your backpack along, filled. If you're new to backpacking in general, start with a lighter-weight backpack at first. Add weight as you get stronger and build your endurance.

If you do not have access to mountains and wild terrain, choose hills and stairs within your neighborhood. Walking up a slight to moderate grade or several sets of stairs with a weighted backpack on can be quite a workout. Start with just one day a week and work your way up to several, depending on how long and how far you plan to hike. If you're planning to go on an extensive backpacking trip, for example, you might want to train this way every other day. If you just want to improve your day-trip endurance, you can probably get away with "weighted" hill training just one or two times per week.

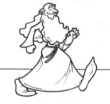

Wise Walkers

Weighted squats and lunges are good lower-body exercises if you're training for hiking and backpacking. Lateral raises, reverse flies, and dumbbell flies are good for your upper-body strength, too. See Chapter 7, "Warming Up, Cooling Down, and Yes! Stretching," for a description of these exercises.

You can also use gym equipment to train for a mountain hike. Treadmills have the capacity to incline, so use them to train for your hikes. The StairMaster can also be used as a training tool for hiking and backpacking if you do not have access to the outdoors. It's especially effective for those more mountainous adventures.

Safety: From Wild Cats to Wild Flowers

Having a fully equipped safety kit is essential for staying healthy during your hikes. Even though the chances of your using anything other than the box of Band-Aids are slim, it is still a good idea to go prepared. Whether you are going for the long haul or just a day excursion, knowing what to expect and being prepared for the worst is a smart move. Most outdoors stores carry first-aid kits equipped with all of the essentials. Ask the clerk for a description of the contents and a brief explanation of how to use each item if you feel the need.

While most plants are harmless, those such as poison ivy and poison oak can cause uncomfortable and sometimes painful reactions. The ivies are the poisonous plants that you are most likely to come across when out in the backcountry. The following are a few tips on avoiding and dealing with the ivies:

➤ Avoid plant contact by wearing protective clothing (lightweight long pants, socks, and long sleeves) when hiking in heavy-growth areas.

Walkers Watch Out!

Needless to say, I strongly recommended that you not eat any wild plant life, no matter what you've heard.

➤ Wash clothes and sneakers that were worn in areas where poison ivy is abundant.

➤ If a reaction occurs—an itchy, blistering rash that is normally in a line pattern—rinse off the area thoroughly, and then apply a topical anesthetic cream or spray, such as Lanacane Maximum Strength First Aid Spray, to help stop the itch without having to touch the sensitive skin.

➤ If you walk with a pup, make sure you wash him thoroughly as well. The oil from poison ivy and oak rubs off on the dog's coat and can then be transmitted to you.

Clubs and Agencies

An abundance of resources is out there with respect to walking clubs and agencies, particularly if you have access to the Internet. Joining a walking club or familiarizing yourself with a walking organization is a great way to get all the latest news on walking and everything that the sport encompasses. My search resulted in sites that offered people anything from training tips for the beginning, intermediate, and advanced walker to great places to hike based on your skill level, location, and desired distance.

Many of the sites I viewed also offered the walker a chance to get involved in the expansion, preservation, and discovery of new and old domestic and international parks and forests around the world. Getting in touch with the expanding world of walking is exciting and invigorating, as it tends to fuel your passion for the sport while giving you a chance to do something positive for the environment as a whole. In Appendix A, "Resources for Walking Fit," you'll find a list of clubs I found useful.

Walkers Without Borders

When you mention the word "vacation" to most people, they think of sleeping late, lazing around, and eating everything in sight. It's payoff for all of your hard work, right? Maybe. But was gaining back all the weight you worked so hard to lose and taking two steps back in your fitness progress really worth it? Probably not. Vacation and gluttony don't have to go hand-in-hand. In fact, in our ever-increasing health-conscious world, more and more people are opting to combine vacation and exercise so they can maintain their fitness while striving for new and exciting experiences (not to mention a little peace of mind).

With the discovery that people are finding pleasure in being active while vacationing, new (and old) companies have started popping up all over the place, offering anyone who is interested the chance to walk rather than bus, train, or fly around the world. Seeing new countries by foot is a much better way to experience different cultures on a more personal basis. Imagine staying in shape while discovering the world! What more can you ask for? For the next couple of pages, we will be looking at what to look for when shopping around for a walking tour. We will also discuss what to bring, as well as some organizations to contact to start you out.

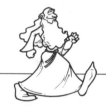

Wise Walkers

It seems that walking with llamas is quite a popular way to hike through the hills, anywhere from Yellowstone to the Smoky Mountains. Go to About.com's "adventure travel" site and look up llama trekking for more information.

Walkers Watch Out!

Backpacking through Europe is fun and cheap, but make sure you are a watchful walker who is aware of your surroundings at all times, and act like you know where you are and where you are going, even if you don't.

Vacation Ventures and Trekking Tours

The best way to ensure a quality walking vacation is to get a referral from someone you know and trust. Asking people in your walking club is another good way to get the upper hand on wonderful walking vacations. If you're not sure, or if you are new to the whole walking vacation circuit, then start out by taking small, shorter trips. This way you can assess the skills and experience of the company without being gone for too long, or putting yourself in danger, or spending too much money.

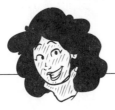

Interesting Excerpts

Adventure travel is a popular trend these days. Vacations designed to educate and involve the traveler in all kinds of fun and "off-the-beaten-track" adventures are a growing fad in the new millennium.

Clubs and Agencies

Agencies that specialize in walking vacations and tours are bountiful, particularly if you have access to the Internet. I searched Yahoo! and found an entire page of domestic and international walking adventures; some offered perks and amenities while others offered challenge and adventure. See Appendix A for some useful resources online and on paper.

The International Volkssport walking clubs in the United States, Canada, Britain, and many European countries have thousands of self-guided permanent trails. Walkers arrive at the starting point, register, take a map, and enjoy the trail, which often includes the highlights of the city, town, park, or area. These are a great way to spice up a visit to any location, or you can plan your entire vacation around them. The AVA Starting Point is a book that gives directions to the 1,100 year-round walks in the United States. You can visit the AVA Web site for a listing of each state and city.

Get Ready, Get Set ... Walk!

So, you've been walking for some time now and you're not only convinced of the health benefits, you're also beginning to realize the many other ways that walking has enriched your life. You've seen all of Europe by foot, joined several walking organizations, helped preserve national trails and parks, and met an entire network of friends and supporters through walking. In addition to completing your third marathon, you've participated in several competitive events that you thoroughly enjoyed. You would like to bring your walking to the next level, but you're not quite sure how. You can't see yourself running, but you don't know what your options are.

Well, how about trying *racewalking*? Racewalking was developed in England over 200 years ago and has been an Olympic sport since 1908. Because it is "low impact," in which one foot is required to remain in contact with the ground at all times, race-walking is much less likely to cause injury than running, but equally as beneficial in terms of fitness challenge. World-class athletes are capable of walking at very high rates of speed, as fast as six minutes per mile. Also, racewalkers get a much better upper-body workout than most runners because of the accentuated use of the back, shoulders, and arms. You burn more calories when you're racewalking because the technique uses more muscles than easy walking, so you can burn as much as two times the calories in the same distance. Finally, you tone your muscles for a sleeker body shape, since racewalking exercises the glutes, thighs, hips, shoulders, upper back, and abs, and it stretches out the muscles for that great long, lean line.

Setting Your Goals

The goal for many racewalkers is fitness. Many, if not most, fitness racewalkers regularly participate in local walks and racewalks to keep themselves fit and on their fitness toes. Many compete for the motivation and challenge. Others race for the fun of it. All are competing with themselves in an attempt to measure the success of their fitness programs through participation in such events. Racewalking goals, like any other goals, need to be realistic, measurable, written down, tracked, and celebrated.

When it comes to racewalking, your goals should be …

➤ **Realistic.** If you are just starting out as a racewalker, make sure you choose an event that is not beyond your fitness level. Since you'll be pushing your pace, you'll want to start with a shorter, more realistic distance first.

➤ **Measurable.** Having a specific, quantitative goal will help to keep you focused and motivated. Registering for an event is a good start.

➤ **Written down.** Writing down your long-term goals, and then breaking them down into smaller, more obtainable ones, is another important aspect of good goal-setting. Planning for an event several weeks ahead of time, and then working your way backward by setting weekly and daily goals, is important.

➤ **Tracked.** Tracking what you do and keeping an eye on your progress will help you decide what works and what doesn't.

➤ **Rewarded.** Rewarding yourself for all of your hard work and efforts will give you incentive to continue to carry on.

> **Weighty Words**
>
> The difference between a **racewalker** and a fitness walker is the state of mind as well as the goals. To be fit is a wonderful goal, and is certainly one worth gaining and maintaining. To be an athlete is to take a psychological step up by creating goals that result in needing the body to change and adapt to complete the goals.

I suggest attending a couple of racewalks as a spectator first. Having an idea of what you are getting yourself into is a good idea. Meeting others involved in the sport is a good way to get some free fitness tips as well.

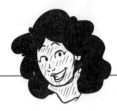

Interesting Excerpts

Most athletes think that the hard days are the most important. But it's the easy days that enable the body to benefit from the hard days, because they provide time for rebuilding to occur.

Training for Events

The principles of training are pretty much the same for every sport. You should follow three general principals. The first principle of training is overload. You must press the body to make the body need to adapt. The second principle of training is specificity. You can't learn to walk faster or more efficiently by taking step or spinning classes. You must do the specific exercise needed to make the desired changes. The third training principle is to balance your hard days with easy days. The "hard/easy" system of training works as well for walking as it does for every other sport. In order for a system to acclimatize efficiently once it's been overloaded, you need to follow with a period of rest and rebuilding. The following table shows some ways to do hard/easy when walking:

Easy	Hard
No walking/alternative activity	Walking
Walking slower	Walking faster
Walking shorter distance	Walking longer
Walking on flat terrain	Walking inclines

Long walks are done to gain endurance, and they are always done at an easy pace. At least one hard day, and no more than three, can be done per week, including speed work and hills. Easy days should usually follow the long days and the hard days like this:

Day	Level	Heart Rate
Monday	Easy	60 to 70% of MHR
Tuesday	Easy	60 to 70% of MHR
Wednesday	Hard	75 to 85% of MHR
Thursday	Easy	60 to 70% of MHR
Friday	Hard	75 to 85% of MHR
Saturday	Easy	60 to 70% of MHR
Sunday	Long walk	

Form

Maintaining proper form during your race is important for two reasons. One, good form helps to decrease your risk of injury. Two, good form makes the difference of whether or not you are disqualified from a race. The leg position, and in particular that of the knee, is one of the most important forms to remember if you want to re-main (qualified and injury free) in the race. Here are some tips that will help you stay healthy and legal:

➤ **Knees:** Straighten knees just before heel contact; don't bend again until behind the body. Be careful of the lead knee swinging too high. This wastes energy and may lead to legality problems. Also, watch out for bent knee on heel contact. This is illegal, as is the lead knee bending before the leg is vertically upright.

➤ **Posture:** Stand tall but not rigid. Stand and do not lean back. The body should be straight and relaxed throughout the entire stride.

➤ **Head:** Hold your head up; don't bury your chin in your chest.

➤ **Shoulders:** Keep them down and relaxed.

➤ **Arms:** Bend elbows about 85 degrees and let relaxed fists arc from waistband to about sternum. Be careful not to swing side to side too excessively as it can throw your center of gravity off and waste excess energy.

➤ **Hips:** Rotate moderately about spine—not side to side; tilt pelvis to minimize swayback. Watch out for excessive hip-drop and excessive lateral hip motion. If the hips move from side to side, the body's center of gravity will move with them. This will slow forward movement and waste energy.

➤ **Feet:** Hold toes up on/after heel contact; roll over feet; toe off; on return to front, let foot skim ground. Be careful not to land flat-footed or with the foot slapping too soon. This has a breaking effect that wastes energy, shortens the stride, and may cause the knee to bend early.

➤ **Stride:** Your stride should be short in front and longer behind. Try to push and not pull, as if walking on a narrow beam.

➤ **Speed:** Increase speed initially by using a quicker step rate; lengthen stride (be-hind the body) later.

Groups to Contact

There are several groups, online and off, with information about racewalking. If you're interested in taking your walking routine to this level, see the section on race-walking in Appendix A.

The Least You Need to Know

➤ Hiking and backpacking are great ways to stay in shape.

➤ Different types of hiking boots are made for different levels of hiking.

➤ Taking a walking vacation is a good way to see the world while staying in shape.

➤ Loads of walking clubs and agencies are available around the world.

➤ Racewalking is as competitive and challenging as running—and just as much fun.

Part 5

Your Feet

Your feet are not only one of the most important parts of your body, they are also one of the least cared-for. For being one of the most essential components of health and well-being, our feet sure do take a beating. High heels, old shoes, poor circulation, and disease are just some of the contributors to the fall of your feet.

Knowing what shoes to wear for walking is a great start toward caring for your feet. Educating yourself on the various types of injuries there are, as well as what kind of treatments are available, is important if you want to keep your feet happy. In this final part of the book, you'll learn the difference between a foot doctor and a bone doctor. You'll discover ways to stretch, massage, and strengthen your feet, as well as how to know when your shoes are wrong for you. Equally as important as burning the calories and building your heart strength is taking good care of your peds, so pay attention as we explore the fun and functional world of your feet.

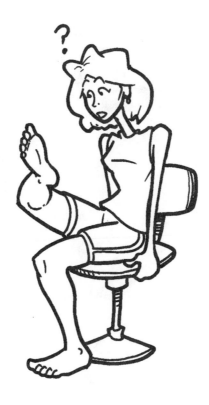

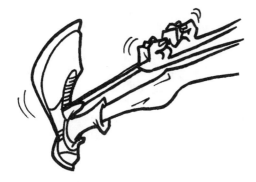

Preparing Your Peds

Once upon a time, athletic shoes were considered unattractive and ungainly. These days, however, a great deal of importance, both in terms of fashion and function, is placed on one's athletic shoe selection. Shoe manufacturers spend a lot of money and time on marketing and research in an attempt to sell their shoes to the masses.

Unfortunately, people get so caught up with the "style" that they lose sight of the function. Choosing the wrong shoe could lead to discomfort, muscle imbalance, and even injury. Knowing what type of foot you have and what type of shoe you need is an important aspect of shoe shopping.

How to Choose a Shoe

Buying a pair of walking shoes involves a lot more than choosing ones that match your outfits. Foot type, walking style, terrain and mileage, arch support, cushion, and shock absorbency are just some of the things to consider when purchasing a walking shoe. And a walking shoe, not a running shoe or a cross-trainer, is what you should be looking for. Shoes are designed to be sport-specific. Walking in a running shoe can

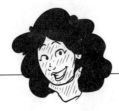

Interesting Excerpts

Nike first created its swoosh logo in 1971 when their shoes were selling for a mere $35.

cause muscle imbalances and other problems, so be specific and choose wisely.

Selecting the proper shoes is crucial for your walking comfort and success. The wrong shoe can cause a whole host of problems, such as injury, muscle imbalance, and lower-back pain, to name a few. But how on earth, given all of your choices, are you to decide what shoe is the *right* shoe? You have to be careful not to get suckered into buying what you do not need. And you needn't spend loads of money on a shoe. Anything over $80 to $100 is unnecessary and somewhat frivolous, and is probably the result of some over-priced marketing scheme. Don't rush into things. Do your research, shop around, and then make a decision.

Foot Type

Our feet generally fit into three different categories. There are the supinators, the pronators, and the neutrals. To find out what category your feet fit into, you can try the wet test. Wet your foot and stand on a dry piece of paper (dark, if possible) and look at the imprint. If the ball and heel of your foot are not joined, or are joined by a narrow band, then you have a high-arched foot, which means you're an over-supinator. On the other hand, if a wide band joins the ball and heel, you have a neutral foot. If they are joined by a really wide band and have little flair where the arch should be, then you have a flat foot and are an over-pronator. Following is a brief description of the three different types of feet:

Pronators: Excessive inward roll of the foot after landing. This twists the foot, shin, and knee and can cause pain in all those areas. Over-pronation causes extra stress and tightness to the muscles, so do a little extra stretching.

You'll have excessive wear on the inner side of your shoes and they will tilt inward if you place them on a flat surface. Knock-knees or flat feet contribute to over-pronation. You should wear shoes with straight or semi-curved *lasts*; *motion-control* or *stability* shoes with a firm, multi-density mid-sole and external control features that limit pronation, are best. Over-the-counter orthotics or arch supports can help, too.

Supination: Insufficient inward roll of the foot after landing. This places extra stress on the foot and can result in iliotibial band syndrome of the knee, Achilles tendonitis, or *plantar fasciitis*. Supinators should do extra stretching of the calves, hamstrings, quads, and *illiotibial* band.

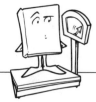

Weighty Words

The last is the section between the insole and the mid-sole in your shoe. If you lift the insole and see a sewn seam, it is a slip last. If you can see a cardboard piece running the length of the shoe, it's a board last. If you see cardboard just at the back of the shoe, it's a combination last. Shoes with slip lasts are more flexible and less stable, while shoes with board lasts are more stable and less flexible. Shoes with combination lasts are a combination of the two.

Your shoes will show wear on the entire outside edge, with the side of the shoe becoming overstretched. Your shoes will tilt outward when placed on a flat surface. High arches and tight Achilles tendons contribute to supination. You should choose shoes with curved lasts to allow pronation. Lightweight trainers allow more foot motion. Check for flexibility on the inner side of the shoe.

To summarize, over-pronaters should look for shoes with straight or semi-curved lasts. Motion-control or stability shoes with firm, multi-density (thick) mid-soles and external control features that limit pronation are best. Over-supinators, on the other hand, should wear shoes with curved lasts to allow pronation. Lightweight trainers allow more foot motion. Check for flexibility on the inner side of the shoe.

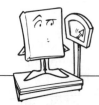

Weighty Words

Motion control shoes are the most rigid shoes. They are designed to be inflexible because they are meant to limit over-pronation. They are generally heavy, but durable. Many are built upon a straight last with the denser material on the inside of the foot to help correct for pronation. **Plantar fasciitis** is a heel spur. The condition is diagnosed with the classic symptoms of pain well-localized over an area of the bottom of the foot near the heel. Often the pain is most severe when you first stand on the foot in the morning.

Neutral-footed people have feet that roll naturally from heel to toe with little excessive movement in either direction. These people can wear just about any shoe that feels comfortable. Adequate cushion for shock absorbency is important. The shoe needs to be flexible enough that the foot rolls smoothly rather than just hitting the ground flatly.

Terrain and Mileage

Two other things to consider when looking for a shoe is the terrain you will be walking on and how much distance you will be covering per week. Terrain can be very different from one route to another. Cement is very hard and can be especially brutal on the joints. Try to buy a shoe that has a lot of cushion for shock absorbency if you're going to be walking on a lot of concrete. If you're an over-pronator, pay special attention to arch support. If you're walking on a sidewalk that is lined with grass, walk on the grassy part as much as possible. If you absolutely *must* walk on cement, put some extra cushioning in your shoe for added support.

Dirt, *Astroturf* (the material most tracks are made of), and grass are much easier on your joints. They offer a natural cushion to help absorb some of the load and impact of your body's weight on your joints. Unfortunately, not all of you have access to softer terrain. It is worth your while to do a little research to find out where your neighborhood tracks are. Finally, try to take your longer walks on dirt, grass, or some other softer surface.

Trails and dirt paths are an excellent, natural surface to walk on, but because of the uneven terrain of trails, you will want to take care to wear extra-supportive shoes. Look for a wide base that isn't too heavy. A shoe that is flexible is important so that your foot can adapt to the variety of surfaces. Some people need extra ankle support because of weak ankles. And, of course, when you are walking on bumpy surfaces you must make sure you pay careful attention to where you are stepping. Falling, stubbing your toe, or tripping over a branch can result in painful injuries. Stop to appreciate your surroundings, but when moving, keep your eye on the road.

Walkers Watch Out!

Old shoes that have been sitting in storage are usually depleted. The glue dries out and hardens, and the soles dissipate. This is why they are on sale! Don't compromise foot health for a good bargain.

The faster and farther you walk, the more wear and tear you'll have on your shoes. Good shoes are built to support the foot and to supply adequate cushion to absorb shock, but they begin to wear down over time. Depleted shoes can cause injury and muscle imbalances. If you're having general aches and pains anywhere in your lower body, including your lower back, but you cannot relate it to a specific injury, you may well need to invest in a new pair of shoes. Make sure you renew your shoes approximately every 500 miles.

If you want to extend the life of your walking shoe (and save some money!), wear it only when exercising and not when you're walking around town. Finally, cheaper brands and shoes on sale tend to lack adequate cushion and support due to shelf life and careless production. So choose wisely and don't be thrifty where your feet and body are concerned.

Shoe Shopping

As I mentioned earlier, it is safer to stick with specialty shoe stores when buying your footwear. A good store will hire and train staff who ideally practice what they preach, and who are walkers or some type of athlete themselves. Before going shopping for your walking shoes, make a list of all the specialty sporting shoe stores in your neighborhood. Call each of them up and try to find out their level of knowledge by asking if they have any good straight-last shoes or good shoes for over-supinators. If they do not answer appropriately or they seem vague, thank them for their time and move on. Keep in mind that a good shoe will cost between $70 and $90. Any more and you are buying style. Any less and it is likely you are getting old, depleted shoes. Also, remember that your athletic-shoe size runs one to one and a half sizes bigger than what you wear for dress shoes. Finally, bring the type of socks that you plan to walk in so you can fit your shoe properly to them. Here are some other guidelines to follow when shopping for a shoe:

➤ If you wear an orthotic, bring it along.

➤ Look for shoes with cushioning for shock absorption, and make sure they bend at the ball of the foot.

➤ Shop in the afternoon, when the feet are slightly swollen.

➤ Make sure the heel is snug and does not slide.

➤ You should have a thumb's width between the longest toe and the tip of the toe box.

➤ Always try on both shoes and lace them as you would for activity.

➤ Walk (or jog) around the store.

Even though most store clerks are not podiatrists or physical therapists, they might be able to give you advice about the right shoe for any type of injury you have. Be as specific as you can about how much and where you will be walking, from terrain to mileage to times per week. Again, be sure to walk around the store for a while and to note any discomfort or irritation. Try on several pairs to compare. Once you've purchased them you can

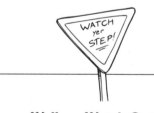

Walkers Watch Out!

Be careful not to lace your shoes up too tight because it can aggravate foot problems as your feet expand during walking.

usually return them, so hold on to the receipt and don't hesitate to return the shoes if you feel you have made the wrong choice.

In Appendix A, "Resources for Walking Fit," you'll find a list of resources that should help you to begin your shoe-shopping adventure. The more you know, the better prepared you will be, lowering your chances of choosing the wrong shoe. Most of these companies have catalogues you can order from, or have phone numbers to call to locate a store near you.

Signs and Symptoms of the Wrong Shoe

Buying and then exchanging the wrong shoe is one thing. Sporting, wearing, and refusing to change the wrong shoe is quite another. As I mentioned earlier, wearing the wrong shoe can lead to a bunch of problems including, but not limited to, lower-back pain, muscle imbalances, foot cramps, and injury. Although you may not be willing to throw away your favorite pair of walking shoes, holding on to them could mean jeopardizing your walking career for days, weeks, and sometimes even months. The American Walkers Association suggests looking out for the following warning signs of a "bad" shoe:

➤ Flared outer soles

➤ Stiff, hard-to-bend outer soles

➤ Flimsy uppers (leather is ideal)

➤ Tight toe box, pressure anywhere on the foot

➤ Slick bottoms (get textured)

➤ Sloppy workmanship

➤ Uneven bottom soles (prominent ridges or rolls)

If your foot swells and feels cramped in the shoe, then you probably need to buy a size or half a size larger. Shoes that don't allow your feet to breathe could aggravate skin injuries like blisters and rashes. If the seams look flimsy and tear easily, then they're probably not made well and you'll have to buy a better pair. Finally, if the shoe is uncomfortable and doesn't feel good on your foot, then chances are you've got the wrong shoe. Happy, snug feet are very important, especially for longer and harder walks.

When to Buy New Shoes

You've never been so happy and neither have your feet. You have found the perfect pair of shoes and they felt great! At least for the first couple months. But you are starting to experience some of the aches and pains associated with depleted and ill-cushioned soles. Is it time to buy a new pair? What if the store doesn't carry your preferred style anymore? Should you just buy three or four pairs of your favorites next time you go, just to make sure you will have a back stock? These are all good questions.

In general, athletic shoes have about a 500-mile or a year's life span, whichever comes first. That is, they are good for 500 miles or a year before the sole and body of the shoe begin losing their protective efficiency. Even if you haven't walked one third of 500 miles, if your shoes have been sitting around for over a year, chances are they need to be replaced. The soles of old shoes dissipate. The glue holding together the base of the shoe dries out and hardens. If you are walking over 20 miles a week on cement, you might want to err on the side of an earlier shoe rotation cycle. If, on the other hand, you are only walking two to four days a week, two to five miles each time, then you're probably safe with holding on to your shoes a little longer.

Wearing Other Kinds of Sports Shoes for Walking

Avoid wearing cross-trainers and shoes designed for aerobics, basketball, or racquet sports. These shoes were designed for a specific purpose other than walking. Shoe manufacturers spend lots of money and time studying the movements of different sports and try to design a shoe that best suits the body mechanics of each sport. Wearing a shoe that was designed for leaping across a wooden court or jumping on and off a plastic step might realign your muscles and bones improperly and lead to injury. Stick with walking, running, and hiking shoes.

Running shoes, on the other hand, are perfectly suitable for walking. If you decide to go with a running shoe, avoid the flared heel. Instead, look for heels that are even undercut at the back to allow for good heel strike and roll through the step. Also, your shoe should not have a high heel and should be no more than an inch higher than the sole under the ball of the foot.

Wise Walkers

Body weight plays a significant role in shoe selection. The heavier you are, the more cushion you will need.

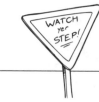

Walkers Watch Out!

Don't stock up on your favorite shoe. Even new shoes get old sitting in the closet for several months in a row. Changes in shoe model from one year to the next have more to do with aesthetics (color and design) and less to do with their actual function.

Sockin' It to Ya

Choosing the right sock is almost as important as choosing the right shoe. What is the point in spending all this time and money on choosing the best shoe when your socks swell or bunch up, causing your shoes to feel tight and uncomfortable? Bad sock choices can cause a lot of discomfort, painful blisters, and even muscle-imbalances by shifting your weight to take the load off sore spots. Factors to take into consideration when sock-searching are finding the right size for your foot, checking for consistency of the texture, and knowing what materials to look for.

The right-fitting socks are very important for walking comfortably. Before you buy your socks, check the label to make sure they aren't going to shrink on you after the first wash. Buy socks that match your shoe size. Buy one pair at a time and try them out; if they work well, go back and buy a bunch more.

The "consistency" of a sock refers to its thickness or thinness. Some people like to wear really thick socks for lots of cushioning and to hold their foot in place. This is fine, but remember that our feet tend to swell as we walk. Tight-fitting socks will only become tighter with time. Consider doubling your socks up if you like that snug feeling. That way you have the option of removing one pair if your feet feel too constricted. Thin socks are less popular than their thicker counterparts, but they do exist. Wearing thin socks is fine, but make sure your shoe fits well. A thin sock and a too-big shoe can cause a lot of chafing, which leads to irritated skin and blisters.

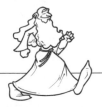

Wise Walkers

Specialty socks are often thick, so they may not fit into your existing shoes. For this reason, try shopping for both socks and shoes at the same time before buying either. If you're a serious walker and you want to take advantage of the latest sock technology, try them on at the same time you fit your next pair of shoes.

The last matter to consider when looking for socks is the type of material they are made of. For a long time people wore cotton because it's inexpensive, easy to care for, and comfy. Unfortunately, cotton does not dry quickly, so you end up walking in damp socks, which have a tendency to expand and cause abrasions. Try a pair of synthetic socks for a trial walk. Good ingredients include a mix of polyester and cotton, or acrylic and cotton. Sports podiatrists frequently recommend appropriately padded socks of acrylic fiber. Acrylic fibers tend to "wick" away excessive perspiration, keeping the foot cool in hot weather. Polypropylene and Coolmax are two notable "wicking" fibers to look for when sock-shopping. ThermaStat is a good fabric for colder weather. Not only does it wick moisture away from the foot so that the foot stays dry, but its hollow-core fibers surround the foot with warm insulating air as well. Most specialty socks are a little more expensive than their comfy cotton counterparts, so don't go overboard and buy a truckload before trying them out first. Try buying a couple of different pairs made of a distinct mixture of materials and try them on for size.

Lacing It Up

I love to run and walk, but if there is one thing that irritates me the most about either activity, it's having to stop to re-lace or readjust my shoe laces, which I do all the time. To this day, I've never managed to tie my shoes "just right." Great shoes and socks are a plus, but feeling like you never really have the lacing "fit" right can be a pain in the … foot, to say the least. The following is a list of foot fallacies and lacing techniques to help:

➤ **Heel slippage:** Loop back through top eyelet to lock the heel in place. Use every eyelet, making sure that the area closest to the heel is tied. When you have reached the next to last eyelet on each side, thread the lace through the top eyelet, making a small loop. Then thread the opposite lace through each loop before tying it.

➤ **Wide forefoot:** Leave the first few eyelets unlaced.

➤ **Narrow foot:** Double back an extra loop or two in the mid-foot to allow for greater tightening. Use the eyelets farthest from the tongue of the shoe. It will bring up the side of the shoe.

➤ **High instep:** Skip all but the very top eyelets.

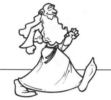

Wise Walkers

Squirt a little water on your shoelaces after you tie them; they should stay tied for the whole day.

In addition, the American Academy of Orthopaedic Surgeons recommends individuals to follow these general lacing tips:

➤ Loosen the laces as you slip into the shoes. This prevents unnecessary stress on the eyelets (small holes for the laces) and the backs of the shoes.

➤ Always begin lacing shoes at the eyelets closest to your toes, and pull the laces at one set of eyelets at a time to tighten. This provides for a comfortable shoe fit.

➤ When buying shoes, remember that shoes with a larger number of eyelets will make it easier to adjust laces for a custom fit.

➤ The conventional method of lacing, crisscrossing to the top of the shoe, works best for the majority of people.

The Least You Need to Know

➤ There are three general types of feet—and shoes made to fit them.

➤ Most shoes are good for no more than one year or 500 miles.

➤ Injury and unexplained pain are likely due to bad shoes.

➤ Good shoes and good socks go hand-in-hand.

➤ Lacing up your shoes correctly will help to prevent foot discomfort.

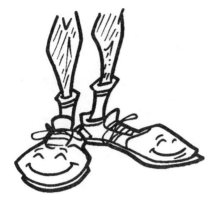

Footloose and Fancy-Free

Believe it or not, we have 26 bones, 33 joints, 109 ligaments, and 19 muscles in each foot, and all of these components work together to enable us to move. You will walk more than 100,000 miles during your lifetime, and may place up to four times your weight on your poor soles. Yet, despite the fact that feet are so important, very few people actually take good care of them. In fact, 75 percent of Americans will experience foot health problems of varying degrees of severity at one time or another in their lives.

Rather than having to take care of your feet once they've been injured, how about watching out for them while they're still well? Wearing the correct athletic shoes is a start, but how about the rest (the majority) of your day? Most dress shoes barely make it in the comfort zone and, with enough time, can cause some irreparable damage. That's why choosing comfortable, functional footwear is key to keeping your feet healthy and happy. In addition, knowing how to realign minor (and major) imbalances using inserts, such as orthotics, is a good way to prevent further damage from occurring. Those are the topics we'll cover in this chapter.

Fashionable Functional Footwear

Quite often, you're forced to make a choice between but uncomfortable feet and ungainly yet contented feet. Bunions, corns, and blisters are just a few of the maladies that some people accept as part of the deal if they want to look good. The American Podiatric Medical Association says that only a small percentage of Americans are born with foot conditions. It's neglect and the lack of awareness and proper care (including poor-fitting shoes) that accounts for most of the problems.

Slowly but surely, however, people are beginning to pay a little more attention and respect to their feet.

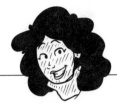

Interesting Excerpts

According to the American Podiatric Association, about 19 percent of the U.S. population has an average of 1.4 foot problems each year. Overuse foot injuries are more common than acute injuries among recreational athletes. Stress fractures, tendonitis, bursitis and plantar fasciiti are just a few of the conditions commonly seen in walkers. Among the causes of these injuries is inappropriate footwear, including shoes that have lost their absorbency, shoes with no arch support, and shoes with overly rigid soles. Walking on hard surfaces and inappropriate stretching are two other causes of overuse injuries.

Shoe manufacturers, both sport and otherwise, have caught on to the trend that having healthy feet means having happy feet, and happy feet means happy customers. Careful engineering and high-tech design, along with special high-end fabrics and cushioning, make up the structure of many of the "comfort" shoes today. In addition, more and more people are realizing the importance of having comfortable, healthy feet all day long as opposed to just during exercise. Wearing shoes that take care of the health of your foot on a constant basis is key to maintaining overall well-being. Anyone who has had a foot injury or chronic foot problem knows how painful, expensive, and time-consuming it can be.

Finding the right walking shoe for exercise took some time and energy, I know. But your feet and back are probably thanking you by now, right? Since you've spent so much time deciding on the perfect walking shoe, why should you compromise your feet by wearing less-than-comfortable shoes during work and play? Your feet need just as much care while you're sitting, standing, or walking to and from your daily doings as they do while you're on the treadmill. Since you've come this far, you might as well go all the way and invest in ways to improve the health of your foot both on and off the track. Besides, what good are great walking shoes when you can't walk because your feet hurt all day from poor dress shoes? In fact, doctors of podiatric medicine believe high heels are orthopedically unsound, and attribute medical, postural, and safety problems to their use.

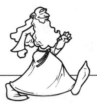

Wise Walkers

Try to decrease the amount of time you spend in heels. Wearing them frequently and for long periods of time may decrease the range of motion in your feet by shortening the Achilles tendon. The Achilles tendon is a thick tendon that connects the calf muscle to the heel. When you wear high heels, the heel is raised, shortening (and tightening) the Achilles band. When you take your heels off and return your heel to its natural position you are stretching the Achilles tendon, causing micro tears, which are healed with scar tissue. Scar tissue is less pliable than the original tissue, which exacerbates the problem of tightness even more.

Shoes must have the ability to protect the foot while enabling you to perform your daily duties without pain and discomfort. The following is a list of "features" to look for in an everyday walking shoe:

➤ **Construction:** Look for solid construction techniques such as tight, well-sewn seams and unyielding transitions where layering is present. This will indicate that some engineering, time, and *pedorthics* has gone into the making of the shoe.

➤ **Materials:** The materials of the shoe should be of good quality, like leather or suede. Synthetic materials such as pleather will not mold to your foot's shape and may eventually cause blistering.

➤ **Heel height:** The shoe should basically be flat-heeled. In a flat-heeled shoe, the shoe and foot generally function together, the heel continues to rise naturally, and the foot gives a normal push-off.

➤ **Shoe shape:** The shoe's shape should match the foot's shape so that function and comfort are both achievable. When a shoe's shape is greatly different than the foot's shape, discomfort and, eventually, damage can result.

➤ **Shoe length and width:** The length and width of the shoe depends on the individual's foot as well as on the activity the shoe is being purchased for. A foot's proportions change, depending on a person's activities, which is why it is important to try the shoe on and to walk around in it before purchasing it.

➤ **Shoe fit:** The fit of the shoe depends on the individual as well as on the manufacturer. The same shoe "size" often differs from one shoe company to the next. Give yourself one half to one inch of room in the front of the shoe for foot swelling. Most importantly, make sure that the shoe is comfortable and that it feels good.

Don't worry—there's no need for you to give up style and fashion for comfort. Again, many shoe manufacturers are taking these factors into consideration. In Appendix A, "Resources for Walking Feet," you'll find a list of some of the companies offering safe and stylish footwear.

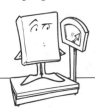

Weighty Words

Pedorthics (pronounced *ped-OR-thix*) is the design, manufacture, modification, and fit of footwear to alleviate foot problems caused by disease, congenital defect, overuse, or injury.

Inserts

Uncomfortable feet are most commonly associated with ill-fitting shoes. But not always. Despite the fact that you've spent time, money, and a great deal of research to find the "perfect" shoe, your feet, back, or knees still hurt. Structural problems like muscle imbalance, misaligned bones, weak ankles, limb-length discrepancies, flat feet, and high arches can lead to a whole host of problems, including but not limited to, back, ankle, and knee pain. Many of these aches and pains are due to maladjustments developed over time from improper gait and limb alignment. Fortunately, foot-care professionals have developed ways to realign these discrepancies by creating something called an insert.

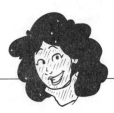

Interesting Excerpts

Foot care has been around for ages, literally. In fact, during the Greco-Roman period, they made attempts to provide artificial prostheses such as wooden legs, iron hands, and artificial feet.

Inserts are foam and rubber pads, gel bags, and premeasured molds that you can purchase to insert inside your shoe to balance out discrepancies such as those just mentioned. Due to environmental (poor shoes) and biological (shape of foot) reasons, many people have had to use inserts to correct misaligned gait and foot-to-ground contact. Years of walking with anatomical dissimilarities such as flat feet, irregular foot sizes, or one limb longer than the other can cause a series of physical compensations that eventually may lead to pain and even injury.

You can purchase several different inserts if you or your doctor has discovered that your gait and body alignment need correction. The most readily available inserts are called insoles; they are made of rubber or are foam fitted for the general public, and are commonly sold over-the-counter. The second type of inserts is called an arch support. Arch supports are designed for the flat-footed individual who needs additional cushioning under their arch. Finally, there are orthotics. Orthotics are custom-made shoe inserts that correct gait problems, provide foot support, relieve pressure on painful areas of the foot, and provide motion control. Talk to your doctor about whether you need orthotics and where to find them.

Insoles

Most shoes, especially athletic ones, already come with an insole meant to provide additional support for the foot. Unfortunately, these "freebies" do not supply enough cushion, shock absorption, or arch support necessary for an "active" individual. Fortunately, many sporting goods and specialty stores sell insoles that provide much more support than those provided by the shoe manufacturer. Insoles come in foam, rubber, gel, and other shock-absorbing material and are commonly sold over-the-counter at most sporting goods and other shoe stores.

Spenco is one of the more common household names when it comes to shoe inserts. Among many things, they make an insole with Rubatex, which offers the foot a "soft bubble" environment for added support and shock absorbency. In addition, their original green slip-in insoles "provide long-lasting heel-to-toe comfort" and are widely popular for those seeking a little extra padding. They also have heel and metatarsal arch cushions to provide support and comfort for the front and back of your foot. Hydropedes is another company that provides cushioning by way of a Glycerine gel-filled insole. This company has designed an insole that moves with the foot, providing the foot with a constant massage, helping to increase circulation, comfort, and general foot health.

Orthotics

Some insoles are constructed to mold themselves to your foot upon wear. These are called orthotics. These are not to be mistaken with custom-made orthotics, which are created specifically for the individual (by using a foot mold) to correct foot and walking problems. These ready-made orthotics are designed to change shape and adjust to your foot's contour after being placed in hot water. Over-the-counter orthotics are less expensive than custom-made orthotics, and may not afford the same degree of relief. These "ready-made" orthotics provide arch support and some degree of gait-correction and cushioning.

Custom-made orthotics are designed to treat or adjust various biomechanical foot disorders, correct gait problems, provide support, relieve pressure on painful areas of the foot, and provide motion control. They are usually prescribed by foot, bone, and health specialists such as doctors, orthopedists, chiropractors, physical therapists, and podiatrists, and are fit by a pedorthist at an orthotics lab. In order to fit you for orthotics, a professional will take a plaster cast of the foot at rest. The orthotic is then constructed to support the foot in that position. Other methods used to measure the feet for orthotics are foam impressions, tracings, or computer measurements. Orthotics are generally grouped into the following three categories:

➤ **Functional orthotics** are designed with special wedges inside them, correcting defects in the arch that cause poor shock absorption, such as excessive pronation or supination. This motion can cause strain on joints and muscles throughout the leg, hip, and back as well as the foot and heel pain of plantar fasciitis.

➤ **Weight-dispersive or accommodative orthotics** typically feature padding designed to relieve pain caused by excessive pressure on the foot and toes.

➤ **Supportive orthotics** are arch supports usually prescribed to treat arch problems.

Several common symptoms may indicate misalignment of the feet and a need for orthotics. If one side of the sole of your shoe wears out faster than the other, your arches are probably either too flat or too high. If you frequently sprain your ankle, you probably have weak ankles or a muscle imbalance, causing instability of the joint. If you have chronic heel, knee, or lower-back pain, your shoes may be the culprit, causing misalignment that affects the balance of the rest of your body. Finally, if your shins or your feet hurt in general, you are probably a good candidate for orthotics.

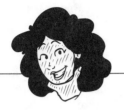

Interesting Excerpts

The American Podiatric Medical Association says the average person takes 8,000 to 10,000 steps a day. Those cover several miles, and they all add up to about 115,000 miles in a lifetime—more than four times the circumference of the globe.

Walkers Watch Out!

Be prepared to spend some money on your custom-made insoles. Orthotics can range from $150 to $400, not including the doctor's visit. Some insurance companies will cover at least a portion of the cost, so make sure you call yours before you buy a pair.

Arch Supports

Arch supports are insoles that are designed specifically to accommodate the arch (or lack thereof) of the foot. People with high arches may have foot pain from walking in shoes without arch support. Similarly, people with flat feet need a little added cushion to prevent excessive stress on the plantar fascia. A ready-made arch support can provide relief and comfort. There are a couple of different types of arch supports. Some arch cushions you can slip into the shoe under the arch, which provide a little extra height. Orthotic arch supports, on the other hand, are ready-made products that conform to your foot shape upon wear, providing a better arch-support fit.

Before you go out and spend money on inserts, I suggest you speak with your doctor first. Have him or her refer you to a podiatrist who can look at your feet from a more professional stance. Many people will buy inserts and wear them incorrectly, only exacerbating their foot problem. A podiatrist will be able to pinpoint the issue exactly and give you advice on how best to approach the problem.

You have a myriad of choices when it comes to orthotics and other special footwear needs. In Appendix A, I provide you with list of specialty stores and manufacturers that I hope you'll find helpful.

Walkers Watch Out!

As you shop for inserts, you'll likely come across products selling the healing value of magnetic inserts. While some believe this type of therapy works, others feel quite strongly that it doesn't.

The Least You Need to Know

➤ Taking care of your feet improves overall well-being.

➤ "Everyday" shoes don't need to be uncomfortable or painful.

➤ Back, foot, and knee pain can be due to misalignments.

➤ Inserts come in the form of arch supports, insoles, and orthotics.

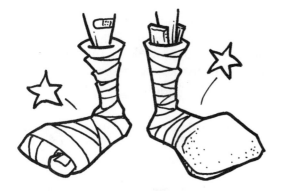

Chapter 23

The Walking Wounded

In This Chapter

➤ There are many types of foot and leg injuries

➤ Knowing the difference between a sprain and a strain

➤ How to avoid blisters and bunions

➤ Over-training can cause injury

Anyone who has suffered an injury knows what a drag it can be. Waiting to recover can be such a frustrating and nerve-wracking experience. In fact, most of us do not have the patience to wait long enough, which is why we end up re-injuring ourselves so often. Giving your body the adequate time and rest it needs to recuperate and re-build is not such an easy discipline to follow. But it is crucial if you want to extend your walking career for months and years to come.

Another common culprit of walking injuries is muscle imbalance and inflexibility. Neglecting to strengthen and stretch your muscles can, and probably will, lead to sprains and strains that, once they have occurred, are difficult to recover from entirely. Spending a little time both before and after your walk to stretch tight muscles and to strengthen weak ones is an important part of a low-injury walking program.

In addition to imbalanced training habits and muscles, we injure our feet through neglect. Injured feet, whether it's from blisters or bone spurs, can put you out of the walking game for weeks. Taking extra care of your feet by choosing the right footwear and practicing proper foot care is essential if you want to continue to walk with comfort and pleasure.

Walking-Related Injuries

One of the many benefits of using walking as your primary fitness is that it's a low-impact sport that puts minimal stress on your body. Constant pounding, fast, jerky movements, and repetitive jumping up and down are all movements that increase your risk of injury. Thankfully, walking does not involve any of these actions and thus remains relatively low on the injury scale. But injury can occur, which is why we must spend some time discussing it.

Most walking injuries have more to do with inappropriate footwear, improper training, insufficient rest, and lack of stretching than an actual incident, such as a fall or twist of the ankle. The *over-training syndrome* and inadequate rest are probably the most common reasons for injuries today. As we have already discussed, many people find it very difficult to moderate their exercise routine once they get going, and so they tend to do too much too soon. Skipping "rest" days is not an uncommon occurrence, especially when you are feeling so good and so strong. Yet, it's during the "rest" days when your muscles and cardiovascular system rebuild themselves. Not having this time to restore itself will keep your body in a constant state of "breakdown," which weakens the muscles and connective tissue and, eventually, leads to injury.

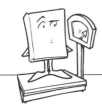

Weighty Words

The **over-training syndrome** is the name given to the collection of emotional, behavioral, and physical symptoms that persist for weeks to months. It is also referred to as "burnout" or "staleness."

Knowing when you're overdoing it is the first step in preventing injury and burnout. Unfortunately, most people have a hard time recognizing the symptoms of over-training and end up injured and not knowing why. The following is a list of signs and symptoms that might indicate that you are overdoing it:

➤ Mild leg soreness and or general achiness

➤ Pain in muscles and joints

➤ Feeling washed out, tired, drained, a lack of energy

➤ Sudden drop in ability to walk "normal" distance or times

➤ Insomnia

➤ Headaches

➤ Inability to relax, feeling twitchy or fidgety

➤ Insatiable thirst, dehydration

➤ Lowered resistance to common illnesses: colds, sore throat, etc.

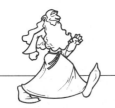

Wise Walkers

As pronation of the foot occurs, the limb above becomes misaligned, which causes increased stress on the muscles on the inside of the foot and leg, and may contribute to greater hip and knee and foot problems.

To play it safe, I suggest scheduling a couple days a week when you perform either very light exercise or no exercise at all. Think of it as an investment, or insurance against your future walking career. You may feel energetic and want to exercise, but give yourself the day off anyway. Beyond maintaining good training principles for your body, it teaches you about discipline for your mind.

As for stretching, people who do not spend sufficient time on increasing and maintaining flexibility are likely to experience some mild form of injury as well. After you exercise, your muscles and connective tissues become tight. By not stretching them out after your walks, you're causing the tighter muscles to pull and strain other weaker muscles.

For example, tight quadriceps muscles will pull on the hip flexor (the muscle in the front of your hip that connects to your spine) and cause stress and strain of the lower back. You might also cause added wear and tear to the joints of your body by not stretching. A tight thigh muscle may pull the kneecap out of line, causing it to rub on the other bones in the joint, which eventually leads to bone degeneration—something that is irreparable.

Wise Walkers

Keeping your body limber and loose will also prevent injuries on the road. Increased flexibility means added agility, and the more nimble you are, the less likely the chance of injuring yourself by losing your balance and falling or twisting an ankle.

Shin Splints

Shin splints are the most common condition new walkers experience, especially if they are trying to walk fast. Shin splints are described as a pain in the lower leg that is due to over-striding, downhill walking, wearing high-heeled shoes, and over-pronation. "Splints" is a term used to describe pain along the shin (tibia) and is commonly seen as an overuse injury. It usually develops gradually over a period of weeks to months, but may occur after a single excessive bout of exercise.

Immediate treatment for shin splints is ice therapy and anti-inflammatory medication such as ibuprofen. Apply ice for 10 to 20 minutes on the sore area, three or four times a day. The long-term treatment for shin splints is rest. Taking several weeks off (if there is pain with daily activities) or just decreasing the amount and type of activity that initially aggravated the inflammation is a good idea. An effective formula is to minimize your walks to a

Walkers Watch Out!

Walkers with shin pain should be aware of a condition called "compartment syndrome," which involves an acute inflammation of the lower leg in which the blood supply is cut off. A lack of blood could cause necrosis (death of tissue) of the affected limb. See your doctor if you are experiencing consistent lower-leg pain with pressure.

50 to 90 percent drop in duration, and doubling or tripling the time between each workout. This "active rest" will enable your body to loosen up and heal. Reinforcing your regular walking routine too soon will likely end up exacerbating your injury even further, so be patient and relax.

Massage is another effective treatment for shin splints. Applying pressure to thick, tight areas within the muscle, to break down lesions and scar tissue, can be helpful and may prevent recurrence. Also, making sure to correct any abnormal biomechanics will help ensure that the problem does not reoccur. Strength training and shoe inserts are common correctional therapies. Focus on your calves in particular. Pointing and flexing the toes against resistance is a good way to strengthen the calf. Balancing on one foot is another effective exercise to strengthen the lower leg, as well. Finally, stretching after your warm-up, as well as after your walk, will decrease the likelihood of recurring shin splints in the future. Refer to Chapters 7, "Warming Up, Cooling Down, and Yes! Stretching," and 8, "Why Weight?" for a description of calf stretches and strengtheners.

Walkers Watch Out!

Every time your ankle is strained or sprained, the ligaments are stretched more. The more your ligaments are stretched, the more likely the ankle will be strained or sprained. The result of this cycle is a permanent instability of the ankle.

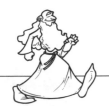

Wise Walkers

A company called Active Ankle sells an ankle support called the T1 that "provides maximum ankle mobility for chronic instability," if you want to take extra care to protect your ankle. They offer other ankle support products as well, at www.active-athlete.com.

Ankle, Knee, and Leg Injuries

Injuries of the leg are not uncommon in walkers, especially since they are the most commonly used (and abused) limbs. Many of the injuries associated with the leg have to do with wear and tear, muscle imbalance, weak connective tissue, or improper footwear. Most of these can be alleviated with rest and ice, while others may require a little more rehabilitation and strengthening. Paying attention to your body is an important factor in reducing your risk of injury. Staying within your program, and not doing too much too soon, will give your body time to heal and make it less susceptible to injury. But some pain is to be expected. Knowing the warning signs and how to distinguish between regular muscle soreness and the beginnings of an injury are important aspects of keeping you safe and injury-free.

The ankle is a very complicated and intricate joint. It connects your leg to your foot and is made up of a complex network of ligaments that hold the joint together. The ankle is one of the most commonly injured joints in the body. Because it is involved in all weight-bearing activity, it takes a lot of abuse. Ankle injuries can range from minor sprains to full-out ruptures. Unfortunately, once you've sprained an ankle, the ligaments never fully heal to 100 percent and are therefore more prone to recurring injury. That's why it's so important to give your injury adequate time to heal as well as to rebuild strength.

Immediate treatment for an ankle sprain involves rest, ice, compression, and elevation (or R.I.C.E.), a procedure that will be explained in more depth in the next chapter. Basically, during the first few hours after an ankle injury you should sit (or lie) down to take the weight off the joint. Apply ice every few hours for 15 to 20 minutes, and then elevate it to keep the swelling down. Wrapping the joint in an Ace bandage will prevent it from moving, since movement could exacerbate the swelling even more.

Once the swelling and inflammation have gone down (which may take several days or even weeks, depending on how severe the injury is), it's recommended that you complete a series of range-of-motion exercises to loosen up the joint and break down the scar tissue. Once the joint, ligaments, and tendons become more pliable you can begin strengthening the muscles around the ankle. Finally, when you feel that your ankle is stable enough, you can return to a modified version of your walking routine. Remember to take it slow during the first two to three weeks after you return to activity. The following is a list of range-of-motion and ankle-strengthening exercises for the ankle:

1. **Plantar/dorsy flexion:** For increased range of motion, point and flex your toes. Repeat 10 times each.

2. **The alphabet:** To increase range of motion, use your toes and foot to outline the alphabet in mid-air. Repeat on the other foot.

3. **Toe raises:** For increased strength, hold on to a chair or support yourself against a wall, and lift your right leg into a hamstring curl (shin parallel to the ground); extend your left ankle and lift your body on the toes. Slowly lower and repeat 8 to 12 times.

4. **Resistive exercises with towel for strength.** Sit on the floor with your legs straight out in front of you. Wrap a towel around the ball of your foot and pull it toward you. As you do this, try to point your toes to resist the movement. Repeat 8 to 12 times.

5. **Balance exercises for strength.** Stand on one leg with the other leg bent, so that the thigh is parallel with the floor. Lower your body slightly if you can, and then come back up. Repeat 8 to 10 times.

The knee is another joint that is commonly the victim of walking injuries. Claimed to be the most vulnerable joint in the body, the knee takes a lot of abuse during athletic activity. Like the ankle, many knee injuries have to do with general wear and tear of the ligaments and other connective tissue, as well as muscle imbalance and lack of flexibility. The most frequent knee injury associated with walking is called chondromalacia, or patella femoral syndrome, which involves the wearing away of the cartilage under the kneecap. Fortunately, because walking is a relatively low-impact activity, the knee does not take as much abuse as running or other high-impact aerobics, so injuries are less common. But they do occur, so it is wise to be aware of what they are and how to treat them.

Because of its bony structure, the knee joint has protective lining known as cartilage, which protects the bones from banging and rubbing against each other. Unfortunately, this protective layer wears down, which leads to painful inflammation as the kneecap rubs against the bones of the femur. Excessive pronation, weak quadriceps muscles, and an imbalance between weak front thigh muscles and tight back thigh muscles, all act to pull the kneecap out of its groove and rub against the bony structure within the knee. Symptoms of chondromalacia include pain beneath or on the sides of the kneecap, swelling, and grinding, as the rough cartilage rubs against cartilage when the knee is flexed. As with the ankle, immediate treatment is rest, ice, compression, and elevation.

Once the pain and swelling are gone, you can begin to perform exercises to strengthen the quadriceps, which will lift some of the weight off the knee. Start with no-weight-bearing exercises like leg lifts with ankle weights, and then move on to a more advanced exercise such as wall sits.

1. **Straight leg lifts:** Begin by lying on your back with the right leg straight and extended; the left knee is bent, with the left foot flat on the floor. Contract the right thigh muscles to straighten (but not lock) the knee. Slowly raise the leg until the knees are parallel, and then lower. Repeat 8 to 12 times, working up to two sets on each side.

2. **Wall sit:** Stand with the lower back against a wall. The feet are shoulder-width apart and a comfortable distance from the wall. Keep the body erect. Slowly bend your knees and your lower body until the thighs are parallel with the floor; keep the knees above (not in front of) the feet, and the abs contracted to avoid excess sway in the back. Pause at the bottom and hold for 30 seconds, and then stand back up. Repeat 8 to 12 times, working up to two sets.

The best way to combat these types of injuries is to make sure you're adequately warmed up before you set out on your walk. You want to feel your heart level rise and your muscles warm. In addition to a sufficient warm-up, you'll want to spend at least 10 to 20 minutes stretching after each walk. Refer to Chapter 7 for a list of warm-up and stretching exercises good for walking.

Sprains and Strains

Sprains and strains are very common in exercisers, especially in beginners who are overweight and in poor condition. Again, tight, imbalanced muscles and over-training are often the culprits. Jumping into a program without adequate time for rest weakens the tendons and ligaments and makes them more prone to injury.

What is the difference between a sprain and a strain? A sprain involves injury to a ligament that supports a joint. Sprains usually occur secondary to trauma (a fall or a twisting injury) and range from a first degree (indicated by the stretching of ligament) to a third degree (described as a complete separation), and can take weeks (and sometimes months) to heal. The individual will usually feel a tear or pop in the joint followed by pain, bruising, and inflammation around the injured area.

A strain involves injury to the muscles and tendons that move the bones of the joint. Strains usually are associated with overuse injuries and refer to a stretching of a muscle or muscle tendon, which can range from a minute tear in muscle fiber to a complete separation of the muscle tendon. Usual symptoms include pain, muscle spasm, muscle weakness, swelling, inflammation, and cramping. Sprains and strains should be treated with … you guessed it: rest, ice, compression, and elevation. Moderate activity can be ensued after the swelling and pain have subsided. Adequate stretching and strengthening are an important follow-up to all sprains and strains.

Blisters and Bunions

Blisters are probably the most common injury known to walkers, and are usually due to ill-fitting footwear. Shoes that are too small or too big can cause friction that may lead to a tearing of the skin. Wet socks or socks that are too big are also common causes for blisters.

Treat a blister by first cleaning it with rubbing alcohol or antibiotic soap and water. Second, you'll need to release the fluid with a needle or pin that you first sterilize by heating it over a flame until it glows red (allow it to cool); you then puncture a small hole at the edge of the blister. Drain the fluid with gentle pressure and then apply an antibiotic ointment, such as bacitracin with polymyxin B (double-antibiotic ointment), or bacitracin alone.

Finally, cover the blister with a bandage and don't forget to change the dressing daily. The best way to

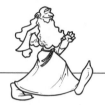

Wise Walkers

A good way to remember the difference between a sprain and a strain is to remember that the latter involves tendons, and that the "t" in strains is for tendons.

Walkers Watch Out!

Once you have suffered a sprain or a strain, the joint never heals back to its original strength. When a joint has been injured, the body repairs it with less pliable "scar" tissue. This causes the joint to become less mobile, decreasing its range of motion and causing minor aches and pains where there previously were none. That's why people so commonly re-injure sprained and strained joints or complain of chronic pain. To avoid re-injury before you go out for your walk, you must spend extra time strengthening and stretching the injured joint.

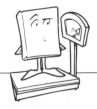

Weighty Words

Bunions are also referred to as Hallux Valgus, in which the joint at the base of the big toe becomes malformed.

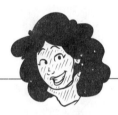

Interesting Excerpts

Plantar fasciitis is most commonly seen in middle-aged men because they tend to wear flat shoes with no arch support, whereas women tend to wear heels which have a little more of an arch. And it's flat feet (over-pronation) that is the leading cause of plantar fasciitis. The condition can also be the cause of sudden weight gain. Rapid weight gain doesn't allow your body and joints to adjust to the sudden extra pressure being exerted on it. Tendons and muscles have to work a little harder to support the added weight, which may cause micro tears and inflammation.

avoid blisters is to invest in comfortable, properly fitting shoes and socks. Refer to Chapter 21, "Preparing Your Peds," for guidelines on choosing the right footwear.

A *bunion* is a malformation of the joint of the big toe due to abnormal pressure or rubbing. Most of the symptoms develop over time when the skin and soft tissue are caught between the hard bone on the inside and the hard shoe on the outside. Any prominence or bump in the bone will make the situation even worse. Shoes that are too small, especially in the toe box, can cause bunions. To decrease the pain, you must eradicate the pressure. Wearing comfortable shoes that allow your toes to move around will alleviate some of the pressure. Sometimes surgery to correct alignment of the toe joint is required if the bunion has grown too large.

Bone Spurs and Plantar Fasciitis

A bone spur is a hard, bony growth and, in most cases with walkers, it occurs in the tissue of the heel. The condition is caused by inflammation of the tissue at the bottom of the foot, known as the plantar fascia. The plantar fascia is a structure that runs from the front of the heel bone (calcaneus) to the ball of the foot. This dense strip of tissue helps to support the longitudinal arch of the foot. When the foot is on the ground, a tremendous amount of force is concentrated on the plantar fascia. This can lead to stress on the plantar fascia where it attaches to the heel bone.

The symptoms of plantar fasciitis include pain in the center of the heel with weight bearing, which is usually most pronounced in the morning when the foot is first placed on the floor. Treatment usually begins with switching shoes to ones with more arch support. Orthotics also have been proven to help with plantar fasciitis. Anti-inflammatories offer temporary relief, along with ice and rest. Avoid weight-bearing activity while recovering from your heel spur. Bike riding and swimming are excellent alternatives until your injury is healed.

Hammertoe and Ingrown Toenails

Hammertoe, or claw toe, describes a condition in which the second toe (which is sometimes longer than the "big" toes) has become crunched from having to fit into a shoe that is too small or too pointed. Because most people buy shoes to fit their "big" toes, they force their second toe to accommodate to the limited space. People who have an exceptionally high arch have an increased chance of developing hammertoe. Again, improper footwear is the culprit here. Selecting shoes and socks that do not cramp the toes will help alleviate aggravation.

An ingrown toenail is a condition that most commonly affects the big toe. Ingrown toenails are commonly a result of excess pressure from wearing improper shoes, as well as lack of care of the toenails. Improper trimming of the nail causes problems such as overgrowth of the tissue at the side of the nail. In the case of the ingrown toenail, the nail groove begins to disappear and the chronic pressure of the nail edge rubbing against the nail groove causes irritation and swelling of the surrounding skin. In addition to investing in some comfortable, properly fitting shoes, you should trim your toenails often. Make sure to trim them straight across and never below the end of the nail groove.

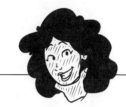

Interesting Excerpts

Overlapping toes are another common foot problem. The condition is usually caused from wearing footwear with a constricting toe box and can be remedied by switching to a pair of shoes with a wider toe box. You may also purchase forefoot supports such as gel toe straighteners, gel toe caps and toe combs to keep overlapping toes apart.

The Least You Need to Know

➤ Improper footwear and over-training are a major cause for injury.

➤ Your first ankle sprain could lead to more down the road.

➤ Being aware of proper body mechanics will decrease your risk of injury.

➤ Trimming your toenails will prevent ingrown toenails.

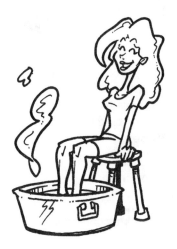

Merry Metatarsals

If you've been injured or have chronic problems with your feet, you might find it difficult to choose what kind of professional help is best for you. You've been to medical doctors for your aches and pains in the past and have heard that physical therapists are trained to treat people recovering from injury, but what about the orthopedists and podiatrists? Where do they fit into the equation? Knowing who's who in the medical world can be quite a challenge, not to mention very confusing. In this chapter, we'll discuss some of the many treatment options available to you and how to know what type of care is best for your particular injury.

Orthopedists: The Bone People

Once known to specialize only in the treatment of skeletal deformities, orthopedists now devote their time to the diagnosis, treatment, rehabilitation, and prevention of injuries and diseases of the body's musculoskeletal system. The injuries that orthopedists treat include arthritis, broken or fractured bones, osteoporosis, sprains, strains, tendonitis, and ruptured discs, to name a few.

Orthopedists are responsible for diagnosing your injury and treating it with medication, exercises, or surgery. They are also in charge of recommending other health professionals, such as physical therapists and fitness professionals, if there is a need to do so. Orthopedists generally deal with more acute conditions that require surgery for injuries to the bones, muscles, and joint tissues, but are trained to provide care for less severe conditions such as sprains and strains as well.

Needless to say, orthopedists encourage physical activity and exercise to help maintain (or improve) your gait, balance, agility, and posture, as well as to enhance other aspects of your health such as your cardiovascular endurance and your circulatory efficiency. According to the American Academy of Orthopaedic Surgeons, exercise is very important for individuals with arthritis and other physical conditions for several reasons. It helps to keep the joints flexible, the muscles around the joints strong, and the bone and cartilage tissue supple and healthy, all factors that minimize your risk of exacerbating the injury and pain.

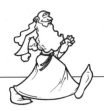

Wise Walkers

If you have a sports or orthopedic injury like tendonitis, arthritis, a stress fracture, or lower-back pain, you may want to consult an orthopedic surgeon who will help devise a fitness routine to minimize the chances of a recurring injury.

Your Local Foot Doctor, the Podiatrist

Podiatrists and orthopedists differ in that the former treats conditions associated only with the lower leg and the foot. Their responsibilities include providing clinical and surgical care for leg and foot problems, with special emphasis on designing custom-made orthotics to correct improper alignments of the feet and legs.

The podiatric physician (doctor of podiatric medicine, or DPM) receives conventional medical training, plus special training on the foot, ankle, and lower leg. Podiatric treatment includes such foot disorders as arthritis, bunions, hammertoe, athlete's foot, foot and ankle injuries, plantar fasciitis, bone spurs, Achilles tendonitis, ingrown toenails, shin splints, and muscle imbalances.

Podiatrists believe in the important relationship between foot health and overall health and welfare. Initial symptoms of such conditions as arthritis, diabetes, and nerve or circulatory disorders can occur in the feet, so foot ailments are sometimes a signal of a more serious medical problem.

But, given the fact that close to 300 foot ailments exist, chances are that your painful peds have more to do with ill-fitting shoes than with some malicious medical malady. Like orthopedists, podiatrists encourage walking and exercise as ways to improve and maintain good health. In fact, the American Podiatric Association says that walking is the best exercise for your feet because it improves circulation, contributes to weight-control, and promotes all-around well-being.

Seeing a podiatrist is probably a good idea if you're planning on starting a regular walking routine. Whether you have foot pain or not, occasional visits to a podiatrist will help ensure that you are maintaining proper muscle and foot balance; an imbalance, if gone undetected, can lead to more serious injuries down the road. In addition, visiting your local podiatrist will give you an opportunity to get some advice on proper footwear and other important walking accessories you might need before you begin.

Marvelous Massages

There is nothing like a good foot massage. Putting your feet up to have them pressed, pulled, rubbed, and stretched is a pleasure like none other. Yet, despite the fact that our feet are involved in almost everything we do, our care of them seems to fall to the wayside. Many people have simply accepted the fact that some foot pain is a part of life and, therefore, to be expected. But ongoing foot pain is not normal and, in fact, can be a sign of some deeper health issues that need to be taken care of. Paying closer attention to your feet will enhance your comfort in everyday life as well as alert you to other health problems that need attention.

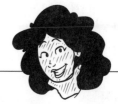

Interesting Excerpts

Did you know that there are close to 13,320 doctors of podiatric medicine practicing in the United States and that approximately 81 percent of all U.S. hospitals have podiatric physicians on staff?

The Indians and Chinese have known the importance of proper foot care since early times. In fact, they were the first to discover a therapy known as reflexology that dealt primarily with massage of the feet and hands. Reflexology is an integrative health science where pressure is applied to reflex areas in the hand and foot, known as *microsystems*, to increase health and overall well-being.

In 1913, Dr. William Fitzgerald, an American ear, nose, and throat surgeon, introduced this therapy to the West. Through application of pressure on particular areas of the hands or feet, he demonstrated that reflexology serves to relax tension, improve circulation, and promote the natural function of the related area in the body. It is a system of massaging specific areas of the foot, or sometimes the hand, in order to promote healing and to relieve stress. You can find your local reflexologist by contacting www.reflexologist.org.

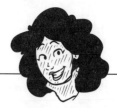

Interesting Excerpts

According to the American Podiatric Medical Association, most Americans log 75,000 miles on their feet by the time they reach the age of 50.

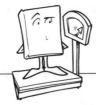

Weighty Words

According to many Eastern medical traditions, a **microsystem** is an area of the body that is a small representation of the whole body. It has been found through thousands of years of experience that the ears, hands, and feet are such areas. According to reflexologists, the more than 7,200 nerve endings in the hands and feet all correspond to some other part of your internal organ system. Thus, when these areas are massaged it promotes healing and health to areas in the body that cannot be directly reached by our hands.

Of course, if the idea of having your feet massaged by a complete stranger makes you uncomfortable, then perhaps learning some tips on how to massage your own feet might be a good idea. There are many different types of massage. For example, there is massage that focuses on *trigger points* and is meant to break down scar tissue and toxins in a particular area in your body. There are soft, relaxing massages meant to calm you and restore energy. There is connective tissue manipulation, trigger-point therapy, zone therapy, and polarity, as well as good old Swedish massage. Although the list is long, let's keep it simple. With respect to your feet, massage is meant primarily to increase circulation, as well to ease minor aches and pains.

Weighty Words

Trigger points are points or areas of pain that appear throughout various parts of the body when a person is not well.

Let's start with your arches. To massage your arches, you will want to use your thumbs. Massage up and down the length of your foot with a circular motion. Use enough pressure to loosen up the tissues and get the circulation going. To massage the top of your foot, grab it by the arch and run your thumb along the top of the foot with a straight line of pressure from top to bottom. Again, don't hesitate to press hard enough to loosen up the tissues. To massage your toes, rub each toe between your thumb, index, and middle finger in a roll motion. Squeeze each toe from base to tip when you're finished massaging it.

Striking a Stretch: A Complete Guide

You all know the importance of stretching your limbs. In addition to releasing tension in the muscles and the connective tissue, stretching increases circulation and blood flow and helps to maintain supple, pliable joints. Getting yourself in the habit of stretching your major muscles was hard enough, and now I'm asking you to stretch your feet? You barely have time to stretch at all, never mind stretching your feet!

Yet stretching your peds is a key factor in maintaining good foot health. Making sure the ligaments and tendons are pliable and strong will reduce your risk of foot and ankle twists and sprains. Increasing your foot's mobility by increasing its range of motion and joint malleability minimizes your risk of accidents and injury. Furthermore, tight muscles and connective tissue in the foot can cause muscle imbalances by pulling your ankle joint out of line, which could eventually alter your foot-to-ground placement and overall gait sequence. A tampered gait will cause muscle and joint to misalign, which, if gone undetected, could end up in structural problems like knee or lower-back pain.

Furthermore, stretching increases the foot's circulation and blood flow, which contributes to better foot health overall. As you can see, spending an extra 10 minutes to loosen your ligaments is a good investment in the future health of not only your feet but your entire body as well. The following are some good stretches for your feet. Do them at home while watching your favorite television show or after your walk with the rest of your stretches.

➤ **Rotations:** Point your toe and flex your foot while you rotate it in one direction. Repeat 10 to 15 times each way.

➤ **Dorsy and plantar flexion:** Point your toe and hold it for five seconds. Then pull your toes back and flex your foot. Hold it for five seconds. Repeat five times with each position.

➤ **Manual foot flexion:** Place your foot over your knee and, using your hand, press down across the top of the foot and the toes until you feel a slight stretch over the top of the ankle and foot. Hold for 10 seconds and repeat.

➤ **Manual foot extension:** Place your foot over your knee, and place the palm of your hand across the ball of your foot and your toes. Using your other hand to secure the foot, press the toes and foot back until you feel a slight stretch along the bottom of the foot.

Walkers Watch Out!

Attempting to stretch cold feet can cause injuries. The best time to stretch your feet is after you've exercised, when the tissues are warm and pliable. Forcing them to stretch when the tissues are cold and unyielding can cause tears in the tissues which may exacerbate injuries when out on the road. To prepare your feet, you can do a few warm-up exercises like toe raises and the alphabet before you proceed with your stretches.

The Healing Touch: When to Use Ice and Heat

I've had several clients ask me what is the proper care for an injury—heat or cold? Some, for example, "swear" that they've heard ice is the best therapy for a sprained ankle, while others claim that they've always put heat on their pain. Confusing? Well, of course it is. But the truth of the matter is, both heat and ice are appropriate treatments for an injury. What is important, however, is knowing when to apply ice and when to apply heat.

An injury, either mild or major, usually involves some sort of tear or damage to a tissue. When this happens, the body responds by flooding the injured area with bacteria-fighting chemicals to ward off infection, and the result is edema, or swelling. This is the body's way of decreasing mobility so as not to cause further immediate damage to the joint. Because heat stimulates blood flow, it promotes healing, relaxes muscles, and eases pain.

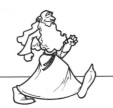

Wise Walkers

Several types of cold treatments are available, including gel pack, chemical bags, ice bags, and ice immersion.

Once the immediate danger of injury has passed, approximately 48 hours, then you will want to start increasing the joint's mobilization in order to remove waste and toxins left over from the edema. Because the injured area is inflated, which may inhibit its range of motion, you'll want to apply ice to decrease the swelling first. This will help to restrict blood flow and minimize the puffiness, which will allow greater ease in moving the joint.

As mentioned in Chapter 23, "The Walking Wounded," rest, ice, compression, and elevation (or R.I.C.E.) are the magic words when it comes to immediate treatment after an injury has occurred. Rest is the first and most important part of care. Taking weight off or discontinuing use of the injured area or joint is the first step. Further immobilization by use of a splint or crutches may be recommended for a short period of time to prevent further injury. Ice application to the injured area or joint, as soon as possible after the injury occurs, will reduce swelling and pain and minimize the inflammatory process. When you apply cold, it slows down the blood flow to the area, reducing swelling and causing numbing of the nerve endings. Once the injured area becomes numb, the cold should be removed. Treatment should consist of 20 minutes of "cooling" (ice on) followed by 20 minutes of "warming" (ice off) for two-hour periods, at least twice a day for the first 72 hours for mild injuries, and longer if more severe.

Wrapping the injured joint firmly with an Ace wrap provides compression. Wear the Ace wrap during periods of activity such as walking, but not while sleeping. Finally, if you elevate the injured part, you'll help reduce pain, swelling, and bruising by draining fluids from the swollen area. The injured area should be elevated during application of the ice and prior to applying compression. Proper elevation has the injured area placed higher than the heart.

Once 72 hours have passed and the swelling has decreased, you can begin your heat therapy—but always under the supervision of qualified medical professional. Heat makes soft tissue more elastic, as well as increasing blood flow, nutrients, and oxygen. It also decreases muscle spasm and joint stiffness. This accelerates the healing process but can also put the joint in a very precarious position. If you administer unsupervised heat treatment, but then turn around and place too much weight on joints that are too relaxed and loosened to handle the load, you could end up injuring yourself even more. Ask your doctor or physical therapist about some information on *thermotherapy*. In addition, here are some different types of heat treatments available to start you off:

1. Whirlpool immersion baths, at 100° to 105°F, stimulate circulation and promote healing of injuries.

2. Hydrocollators—heating pads—provide moist heat, which is more beneficial than dry heat because it penetrates deeper and increases blood supply to the area, and it relaxes the muscle.

3. Ultrasound is the most effective way to achieve deep heat in tissues to help relieve pain and inflammation. It helps to reduce muscle spasms, as well as increase range of motion. Ultrasound is commonly used with conditions such as tendonitis, bursitis, sprains, and strains.

Walkers Watch Out!

You will experience the following sequence of sensations as you begin icing: cold, stinging, burning, and, finally, numbness. Always place a cloth, such as a thin towel or washcloth, between the ice and skin to prevent frostbite.

To Move or Not To Move

The other question I'm often asked when it comes to recovering from an injury is, "Can I move or should I remain immobilized until my injury heals?" Back in the old days, people were encouraged to sit as still as they possibly could so as not to interrupt the injured joint. Images of cast-wrapped individuals with their legs hanging from strange contraptions, bedridden and helpless, have only recently been replaced with something called "aggressive rehabilitation."

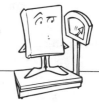

Weighty Words

Thermotherapy is another term for heat treatment.

Aggressive rehabilitation gets the injured party involved in some type of movement almost immediately after the injury has occurred. The idea behind aggressive rehabilitation is to promote tissue healing, blood oxygen flow and nutrition in order to stimulate re-growth and rejoining of disrupted tissues, as well as to prevent *adhesions*. That which was thought to protect the joint in olden days was later discovered to lead to worsened injury, as the impaired tissues became weaker and stiffer with each moment of immobilization. In fact, it was later discovered that prolonged immobilization may cause a 20 percent loss of muscle strength per week, while ligaments may lose 40 percent of their strength.

To avoid this disaster from happening, the Continuous Passive Motion (CPM) machine was invented. The CPM machine rehabilitates the injured area while the person is still recuperating, by moving the joint passively through a modified range of motion in order to stimulate joint motion and increase nutritional input while removing toxic waste. Once the individual is able to move his or her own joint, they proceed with a series of range of motion, flexibility, and strength exercises on a weekly basis. Active exercise during recovery breaks down fibrous scar tissue and increases body temperature and circulation, which removes damaged cells and repairs tissues.

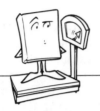

Weighty Words

An **adhesion** is an abnormal union of separate tissue surfaces by new fibrous tissue, resulting from an inflammatory process. Adhesion is often confused with the term abrasion, which is described as a scrape of the top layer of the skin due to sliding or falling against a rough or hard surface. Abrasions are not as serious as adhesions and can be treated by cleaning them out with cold water and an anti-bacterial cream and then covering them with a nonadherent gauze.

The Least You Need to Know

➤ Orthopedists treat conditions involving your bones and joints.

➤ Podiatrists take care of issues with the feet only.

➤ Massage and stretching can contribute to fewer injuries of the foot.

➤ R.I.C.E. is the best "immediate" treatment for most foot, ankle, and knee injuries.

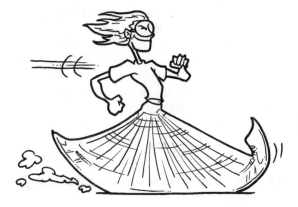

Chapter 25

Walking Wonders

In This Chapter

➤ Learn about the evolution of walking

➤ Who is the fastest walker in the world?

➤ Why walking for a cause is worth it

➤ The longest recorded walk in history

Whatever the reason you've chosen to walk, I'm sure it's a good one. Whether you were inspired by a friend to lose weight, encouraged by your doctor to improve your health, or motivated to discover the beauty of Mother Nature around you, your decision to walk is the right one.

In fact, people have been making the wise resolution to walk for many years. It began as a necessity to help us get around while giving us the ability to use our hands some four million years ago, and has since evolved into one of the world's most popular athletic pastimes. Nowadays, people use walking as a means to lose weight, get healthy, see the world, or spread the word about something important to them. In this final chapter, you'll discover when walking became official and how it has changed throughout the years. You'll also learn about those who have taken the sport to its extreme levels of competition, as well as others who have used it as a means to fight for a cause they believe in.

Historical Moments

Let's face it: Walking has been around, well, forever, really. Or at least for over four million years, ever since the Australopithecus anamensis started walking on two feet, anyway. It wasn't until 100 B.C.E., when Emperor Hadrian ritually toured the Roman Empire, that distance walking was recorded. Hadrian kept the record for many centuries, until Sir Robert Carey walked 300 miles from London to Berwick on a bet. King Charles II didn't take long to catch on to the walking craze when he racewalked from Whitewall to Hampton Court, in the first "racewalk" in history. Then came these crazy "centurions," who challenged themselves to walk 100 miles in 24 hours. The first centurion walk is documented to have taken place in 1762 and was completed by a John Hague in 23 hours and 15 minutes.

The 1800s proved to be a bit more ambitious as a German by the name of Johann Gottfried Seume walked from Germany to Sicily and back in two years. Captain Robert Barclay challenged Mr. Seume's accomplishment by walking 1,000 miles in 1,000 hours; not very speedy at a mile an hour, mind you. This started the "Pedestrian Age" (1860–1903), during which walking became the leading sport in both Europe and America, and was the highest paying, too. In fact, in 1867 Edward Payton Weston walked from Portland, Maine, to Chicago, Illinois (1,326 miles), in 25 days, earning $10,000, which at the time was a lot of money—the equivalent of a million dollars today.

At first primarily a man's sport, walking became popular among women in 1877 when Mary Marshall walked 50 miles in 12 hours. This was followed two years later with the first women's six-day walking race, in which $1,000 was allotted to the first woman to complete the 372-mile distance.

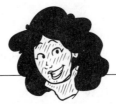

Interesting Excerpts

Edward Payton Weston, "the father of modern pedestrianism," appeared to be the dominating walking figure of the nineteenth century because he walked from Boston to Washington, D.C., for the inauguration of 1860. Seven years later Weston walked from Portland, Maine, to Chicago, Illinois (1,326 miles). Weston's winning streak ended in 1874 when Daniel O'Leary broke his record of 500 miles in six consecutive days and became "Champion Pedestrian of the World." These competitions mark the beginning of the Astley Belt Races which in 1879 awarded Charles Rowell $50,000 in two 6-day races.

The Olympics joined in the fun in 1908, when the British added the 20K and 50K racewalks to their existing list of competitive walking events. Apparently, the Americans liked the idea of fast walking as well and, in 1911, held the first U.S. racewalk on Coney Island. More than fifty years later, the International Volkssport Federation was formed in 1968 to promote noncompetitive walking events, later to be called *volksmarches*. Two years later, in 1970, the First March of Dimes was held in Columbus, Ohio.

Fastest Feet

Currently, walking is one of the most popular forms of exercise in the United States, with 65 million regular walkers. It rises above most other forms of sport and exercise due to its relatively low learning curve and injury rate. It is also very popular because it is highly accessible and can be done anywhere at almost anytime. Walking is becoming a very respected sport, too, as racewalkers and marathoners are breaking new world records for pace and distance every year.

Since the completion of the 2000 Olympic games in Sydney, race times and distances are all the talk these days. I'm not sure about you, but I felt incredibly inspired and motivated by the competition this year, and found myself glued to the television even though it was waaay past my bedtime. I was particularly riveted by the track-and-field events where the mere sight of the physiques of these athletes made me want to get up and go out for some exercise despite the fact that it was dark and late. Just watching these fitter-than-fit Olympiads compete against each other for the gold was enough to convince me that aspirations and dreams are attainable if you just put your mind to it.

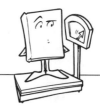

Weighty Words

Volksmarch, also termed volk-swalk, is a walking event. The name started in Germany where these events were originally termed Volkswanderung, or "volkswandering."

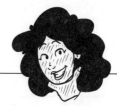

Interesting Excerpts

In almost all of the competitive events I reviewed, I found that men beat women in time and distance across the board. Greater strength and levels of testosterone, among other things, account for the difference.

Although chances are that most of you are not "going for the gold" as it were, you each hopefully have your own dreams and goals to aspire to. If you were lucky enough to share in some of the fun of the Olympics, then you probably know what "inspiration" feels like. Here is a recap of some of the walking victories in the Olympic games in Sydney this year, as well as a list of the world record titles in track and road racewalking to this day:

Year	Country/Gender/Name	Dist.	Time	Rank
2000	China/F/Liping Wang	20K	1:29:05.00	Gold
2000	Polnd/M/Korzeniowski	20K	1:18:59.00	Gold
2000	Nrwy/F/Platzer	20K	1:29:33.00	Slvr
2000	Mex/M/Hernandez	20K	1:19:01.00	Slvr
2000	Spain/F/Vasco	20K	1:30:23.00	Brnz
2000	Russ/M/Andreyev	20K	1:19:27.00	Brnz
Male				
1990	Russ/M/Grigaluinas	1 mi	5:36:09.00	Wld
1989	Italy/M/Benedictis	2 mi	11:47:00	Wld
1979	Mex/M/Colin	10 mi	1:05:07:00	Wld
1990	Plnd/M/ Korzeniowski	5K	18:21:00	Wld
1999	Guat/M/Martinez	20K	1:17:46.00	Wld
2000	Russ/M/Spitsyn	50K	3:37:26.00	Wld
Female				
1991	Italy/F/Salvador	1 mi	6:19:31.00	Wld
1993	Italy/F/Salvador	2 mi	13:23:04.00	Wld
1989	Aus/F/Saxby	5K	20:25:00	Wld
2000	Russ/F/Gudkova	20K	1:25:18.00	Wld
1995	Frnc/F/Boufflert	50K	4:41:57.00	Wld

Wise Walkers

If you're like most Americans, you weren't disciplined in the metric system. Here is a breakdown of miles and kilometers: 1 mile = .621 kilometers, 5 kilometers = 3.1 miles, 20 kilometers = 12.42 miles, and 50 kilometers = 31 miles.

Unfortunately, Americans have not "mastered" race-walking enough to earn a medal or place high in the world rankings, but we seemed to come through in some of the speedier, shorter events to make up for it. Just the same, no matter where these athletes are from, their feats are to be honored and admired. Knowing the hours and hours of physical, mental, and emotional training that goes into just getting yourself out there three days a week, imagine what these athletes went through to accomplish what they did.

Farthest

Finding records for the person who has walked the farthest to date was difficult because records are being broken all the time. I found several stories featuring various individuals traipsing the world, covering thousands upon thousands of miles. Each of their stories was unique and impressive, each pushing the boundaries of distance (so to speak) more and more. Thus, I chose to pick some of the stories that impressed me the most, including a group of Australian 100-mile walkers, called the centurions, who make it their mission in life to cover 100 miles as quickly as possible.

The Australian Centurions was formed in 1971 to honor the feat of those athletes who walked 100 miles within 24 hours on Australian shores. Anybody who can walk 100 miles within a 24-hour time period automatically becomes a lifetime member of the club. The title for the youngest centurion belongs to Bill Dyer who, at the tender age of 16, completed his first 100 miler. Merve Lockyer became the oldest Australian centurion at the ripe old age of 65, having started exercise after a heart attack some years earlier. Chris Clegg has competed in five centurions internationally, including England, Australia, the U.S., and Holland. Ian Jack of Melbourne holds the Australian record for walking 100 miles in 17:59:30 in 1979. Carol Baird holds the women's record for 100 miles in 22:16:43, completed in 1999.

Indeed, it's important to keep in mind that, just because men appear to have broken and dominated many of the walking records, women hold a place in this special history. For instance, at 16 years of age, Ailing Xue of China broke the 20km world record for her age group by completing it in 1:33:10 minutes in 1995. Meanwhile at 2 years shy of 40, Australian Kerry Saxby walked the same distance in 1:31:18 in 1999, winning the world title for the 20k distance in her age group as well.

Australians aren't the only people crazy enough to walk 100 miles in 24 hours. Christina Elsenga of the Netherlands wanted to get in on the fun, and she walked 100 miles on June 6 and 7, 1998, finishing 22nd in 23 hours, 34 minutes, and 17 seconds. She writes about her experience on walking. about.com. Check it out for an entertaining story of mind over matter. It's a good resource for motivation and inspiration.

Wise Walkers

If you walked 1,440 minutes in a 24-hour period, you'd be walking an average of 14- to 15-minute miles. You would walk four miles an hour, which is one mile every 15 minutes.

Dave and John Kunst, two brothers from Waseca, Minnesota, left home with a pack mule they named Willie, on June 20, 1970, to march across the globe. On October 5, 1974, Dave returned home, becoming the first person verified to have circled the earth on foot. The brothers started out by walking from Waseca to New York City to "touch" the Atlantic Ocean. They then flew across the Atlantic Ocean to Lisbon, Portugal, where they again "touched" the Atlantic Ocean, but this time on the other side. David continued on without his brother John as he walked across Europe and Asia to Calcutta, India, where he met up with the Indian Ocean. He then flew across the Indian Ocean to Western Australia. Walking across Australia to Sydney, he touched the Pacific Ocean. From there Dave flew across to Los Angeles, California, where he met up with the Pacific Ocean again. He then walked from Newport Beach,

California, back home to Waseca, Minnesota, in 1974. The walk took four years, three months, and 16 days. Dave wore out 21 pair of shoes, and walked more than 20 million steps and 14,450 miles during his trip.

Dave Kunst, also known as Earth-Walker, paid a painful price for his title as the first man to circle the globe. His voyage put him in the 1997 Guinness record book as well as the 1990 and 1991 *Guinness and Sports Records Book*. He was also featured in the *Ripley's Believe It or Not!* as the "first man to walk around the world." He is now living in Hawaii with a woman he met and married while on his trip.

Good Cause

Walking for the benefit of your own health is a perfectly good cause in itself. Lowering your risk of heart disease, high blood pressure, and other medical conditions can save you and your family from the pain of disease and early death. While most people are motivated by the goal of achieving health and well-being for themselves, some people prefer other reasons to motivate themselves and give meaning to their weekly walks.

Walking to raise money for cancer research, care of AIDS patients, or some other cause is a noble gesture as well as an excellent way to get and stay focused. Many people who "walk for a cause" have personal experience (either directly or indirectly) with the event for which they are walking. Other people like to use their time wisely by practicing good health while contributing to improving the health of others. Whatever the reasons may be, walking to help support some "cause" outside of yourself is a great idea, not to mention an inspirational motivator. Refer to Appendix A, "Resources for Walking Fit," for a list of some good organizations sponsoring walking events that raise money for charity.

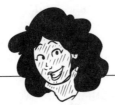

Interesting Excerpts

Theresa del Rosario crossed the Americas in an effort to increase awareness of women's and children's right to good health and safety. The voyage took her two years from the time she left Anchorage, Alaska, on May 12, 1996, to her return on March 9, 1998. Theresa made it all the way to the tip of South America where she landed in Buenos Aires and then turned around and went back. Of the trip, Theresa says: "This journey has been one of trust and respect: of myself, others and the natural wonders around."

Your "quest" for walking doesn't have to be historical, record breaking nor inspired by a good cause. Just taking better care of yourself is awesome enough. The better you feel physically, the better you feel mentally and emotionally, which will not only affect you, but everyone you come in contact with.

In closing, I would like to say that my work as a fitness enthusiast and as a fitness professional has taught me that the line between mind and body disappears rapidly as we become more in tune with our overall health. It makes sense that many of our emotions, as well as our general mental outlook, are a result of how we feel physically. Yet, sadly, many people neglect the needs of their bodies in exchange for success in the professional and financial realms. Hours spent indoors and in cars with poor dietary habits and virtually no physical activity has led to a host of life-threatening medical conditions associated with our increasingly sedentary lifestyles. Unfortunately, warnings of future consequences have not been intimidating enough to encourage people to change their habits until, of course, it's too late.

For this reason, I urge you to take action now. I have discussed the many benefits of walking and exercise throughout this book and encourage you to start thinking about ways you can change your current habits to incorporate more activity into your life. Young or old, slim or plump, fit or not, everyone can benefit from more physical activity, if not for the benefit of our hearts then for the benefit of our minds. All you really have to do is to move more and to remember that every little step counts (literally and figuratively). So good luck and happy walking!

The Least You Need to Know

➤ The fastest mile walked took just over five minutes.

➤ Humans went from all fours to two feet around four million years ago.

➤ Walking became a popular sport in Europe in the 1800s.

➤ You can find many good causes to walk for.

➤ The farthest walk recorded is still going on at just over 34,000 miles.

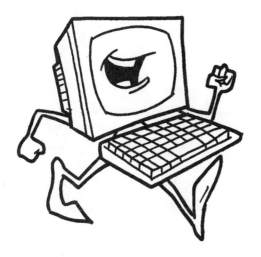

Resources for Walking Fit

Apparel

Champion
5 New England Dr.
Essex, VT 05452
1-888-301-5151
www.championforwomen.com

Champion has a site specifically for women looking for supportive but comfortable active wear. They carry intense- to moderate-activity motion-control sports bras and compression bottoms for women of all shapes and sizes.

Nike
One Bowerman Dr.
Beaverton, OR 97005
1-800-806-6453
www.nike.com

An all-inclusive site that sells the latest trends in shoes and athletic apparel.

RaceReady Clothing Catalogue
PO Box 251065
Glendale, CA 91255-1065
818-547-6869
www.raceready.com

This company offers a large variety of running and walking apparel, including shorts, tops, tights, and warm-up jackets. Their materials are made out of technically advanced fibers such as CoolMax, ThermaStat, Lycra, and Supplex.

Road Runner Sports
Customer Service
5549 Copley Dr.
San Diego, CA 92111
1-800-636-3560
www.roadrunnersports.com

Claiming to be the world's largest running Web site, Road Runner Sports has everything from apparel, shoes, activity logs, and fitness calculators to shoe critics and injury advice. You name it, they've got it.

Title Nine Sports
5743 Landragan St.
Emeryville, CA 94608
1-800-609-0092
www.title9sports.com

A site created by women for women. They carry a large variety of products, including sports bras, jackets, shorts, T-shirts and tank tops, vests, underwear, and much, much more. They cater to the needs of women in particular.

Equipment

Perform Better
M-F Athletic Company
PO Box 8090
Cranston, RI 02920
1-800-556-7464
www.performbetter.com

Perform Better carries products for functional training and rehabilitation. They offer items such as medicine balls, stability balls, rubber tubing, aquatic supplies, heart rate monitors, and mats. They also have informative tips on strength and cardiovascular training, balance, proprioception, and more. They are a small company committed to educating their customer in functional conditioning and rehabilitation.

The Gym Ball Store
16776 Bernardo Center Dr., Suite 101
San Diego, CA 92128-2558
1-800-393-7255
www.physioballs.com

A complete store that offers a wide variety of physio- and medicine-ball equipment and accessories as well as instruction videos and manuals for each.

Polar Electro, Inc.
Heart Rate Monitors
370 Crossways Park Dr.
Woodbury, NY 11797-2050
1-800-227-1314
www.polarusa.com

Polar features an informative site that, in addition to offering you any and all kinds of Heart Rate monitors imaginable, provides information on finding your target heart rate zones, as well as coaching tips and links to events and races.

SPRI
1026 Campus Dr.
Mundelein, IL 60060
1-800-222-7774

Order a SPRI catalogue and receive a plethora of choices in resistance equipment such as rubber tubing, gym balls, weighted bars, and ankle and wrist weights, as well as videos and books on instruction and education.

Whistle Creek Walking Sticks
PO Box 580
Monument, Colorado 80132
719-488-1999
www.whistlecreek.com

The "largest maker of rustic walking and hiking sticks in the United States," they feature 30 styles to choose from, including materials such as hickory, sassafras, oak, pine, aspen, walnut, and cedar.

Treadmills

Precor USA, Inc.
20001 N. Creek Pky.
PO Box 3004
Bothell, WA 98041-3004
1-800-786-8404
www.precor.com

Precor features a wide variety of exercise equipment, including a complete line of treadmills that have won numerous awards such as "Best treadmill judged by personal trainers," the American Council on Exercise award for "Excellence in Customer Satisfaction," and "Highest in overall walker quality, regardless of price." The site also offers suggestions on where to buy comparable products and brochures.

True Fitness
865 Holf Rd.
O'Fallon, MO 63366
1-800-426-6570
www.truefitness.com

Exercise equipment featuring special consideration in evaluating and choosing a treadmill for your home.

Unisen, Inc.
14410 Myford Rd.
Irvine, CA 92606
1-800-228-6635
www.startrac.com

Shoes

Birkenstock
PO Box 6140
Novato, CA 94948.
www.birkenstock.com

A German company known for its high level of comfort and quality with its innovative cork sole, Birkenstock is dedicated to creating shoes that contour to the foot's natural curvature while offering an array of built-in arch supports and other special comfort features.

Dansko
1-800-326-7564
www.dansko.com

Accepted by the American Podiatric Medical Association, Dansko has a wide variety of occupational, leisure, and dress shoes; sandals; and clogs.

Eastbay
111 South 1st Ave.
Wausau, WI 54401
1-800-826-2205
www.eastbay.com

Eastbay is a complete online/catalogue sports apparel, equipment, and shoe-shopping store. They feature 18 different walking shoes with name brands such as Adidas, Nike, Saucony, Rockport, Reebok, and New Balance.

Ecco Shoes
www.eccousa.com

Awarded the "Danish Company of the Nineties," Ecco Shoes uses advanced technology to design leisure and sports shoes to fit your foot anatomically correct in order to achieve the best fit possible.

Fleet Feet
1-800-733-1624
www.fleetfeet.com

Fleet Feet has 36 different locations in the United States and focuses primarily on running shoes and apparel.

Just for Feet
201-760-5000
www.feet.com

In 1998 alone, over 12,000,000 pairs of shoes were purchased from Just for Feet. Their success, in part, is due to being able to serve the needs of a large customer base and offer a huge variety of shoe types and brand names.

Mephisto
305 Seaboard Lane, Suite 328
Franklin, TN 37067
1-888-948-7463
www.mephisto.com

A French footwear company that has a variety of dress and casual shoes with uniquely constructed latex and cork foam footbeds mounted on pure rubber and latex soles to give the most comfortable and durable foot support imaginable.

On Line Shoes
6601 220th St. SW, Suite 10
Mountlake Terrace, WA 98043
1-800-786-3141
www.onlineshoes.com

"Our specialty is walking, hiking, athletic, dress, and casual footwear products. We sell only the best products from the best manufacturers. It is important to us that the footwear you purchase from onlineshoes.com meets your expectations and satisfaction."

Rockport
220 Donald Lynch Blvd.
Marlborough, MA 01752
1-800-762-5767
www.rockport.com

Rockport became the first company to use advanced materials and technologies in traditional shoes to create lightweight comfort. The company features men's and women's dress, casual, and athletic footwear engineered for the biomechanics of walking. Rockport received the American Podiatric Medical Association's (APMA) Seal of Acceptance in 1984.

The Walking Company
9453 Owensmouth Ave.
Chatsworth, CA 91311
1-800-733-1624
www.walkingco.com

The Walking Company is "dedicated to bringing you the finest the world has to offer in technically advanced men's and women's comfort footwear" including a selection of dress shoes as well.

Special Population

American Diabetes Association
1701 North Beauregard St.
Alexandria, VA 22311
Voice toll-free: 1-800-DIABETES
Voice: 703-549-1500
1-800-232-3472
www.diabetes.org

The American Diabetes Association aims at the prevention, improvement, and cure of those suffering from diabetes. The site offers information on nutrition, exercise, grocery shopping tips, communities, publications, and education.

The American Dietetic Association
216 West Jackson Blvd., Suite 800
Chicago, IL 60606-6995
Voice toll-free: 1-800-366-1655
Voice: 312-899-0040
www.eatright.org

This is an organization that is committed to bettering the health of the American people. They offer healthy lifestyle tips, a complete nutritional guide, links to a knowledge center for educational advancement, as well as access to meetings and events.

American Heart Organization
7272 Greenville Ave.
Dallas, TX 75231-4596
Voice toll-free: 1-800-242-8721
Voice: 214-706-1552
www.americanheart.org

As the "official Web site for the American Heart Association" this site offers a surplus of information on anything and everything that has to do with strokes and heart disease. This includes, but is not limited to, risk assessment, dietary and exercise guidelines, advocacy, and legislation, as well as education and a complete reference guide.

Arthritis Foundation
1330 West Peachtree St.
Atlanta, GA 30309
404-872-7100 or 1-800-283-7800
www.arthritis.org

The goal of the foundation is to help find a cure, prevention, or better treatment for arthritis. This includes offering services such as self-help courses, instructional video-tapes, list of support groups, educational brochures, funding, and more to those affected by arthritis.

Gentle Fitness
732 Lake Shore Dr.
Rhinelander, WI 54501
1-800-566-7780
www.gentlefitness.com

This is a resource that offers fitness videos and tips for those suffering with special medical conditions such as fibromayalgia, Parkinson's, arthritis, stroke and cardiac rehab, cancer, Lupus, diabetes, and more. It blends yoga, t'ai chi, and Feldenkrais with today's state-of-the-art exercise physiology and kinesiology for a complete routine to help you sleep better, improve balance, and functional capacity, and relieve pain.

National Diabetes Clearinghouse
1 Information Way
Bethesda, MD 20892-3560
301-654-3327
www.niddk.nih.gov/health/diabetes/ndic.htm

This resource offers a variety of information on diabetes including responses to inquiries and publication references.

National Institute of Arthritis and Musculoskeletal and Skin Diseases/NIH
Bldg. 31/Rm. 4C05, 31 Center Dr., MSC 2350
Bethesda, MD 20892-2350
301-496-8190
TTY: 301-565-2966
Fax: 301-480-2814
www.nih.gov/niams

NIAMS is a useful resource for those suffering from diseases of the bones, joints, muscles, or skin. The site offers a list of fact sheets and brochures as well as clinical reports, health statistics, and informative resources.

Outdoor Adventures

American Hiking Society (AHS)
1422 Fenwick Lane
Silver Spring, MD 20910
301-565-6704
www.americanhiking.org

The AHS is an alliance of hiking organizations, news, and resources, as well as trail conservation and policy.

The Countryman Press
W. W. Norton & Company, Inc.
500 Fifth Ave.
New York, NY 10110
212-354-5500
E-mail: CountrymanPress@wwnorton.com

This company publishes books on rural life, regional travel, nature, and outdoor recreation.

Great Outdoor Recreation Pages
22 West 19th St., 8th Floor
New York, NY 10011
1-800-784-9325
www.gorp.com

The Great Outdoor Recreation Pages has a complete list of hikes and backpacking trips as well as weekend getaways.

Hike Net
Tom Caggiano
275 Route 10 East, Suite 220-237
Succasunna, NJ 07876
Fax: 973-927-3484
www.hikenet.com

This site has one of the world's largest listings of hiking and outdoor clubs in the United States and internationally.

www.peaktopeak.com
Features a list of national parks, state parks, and forests, as well as links to commercial and international outdoor sites.

Walking Adventures International
PO Box 871000
Vancouver, WA 98687-1000
1-800-779-0353

Introduces walkers to the history and culture of the areas through which they are traveling. They also provide travelers with memories and pictures of the scenic highlights of the lands they are visiting. Clients are in the company of ordinary, local walkers, and are guided by a competent, caring member of their Walking Adventures family.

The Walking Connection
4722 W. Continental Dr.
Glendale, AZ 85308-3440
1-800-295-WALK
www.walkingconnection.com

Offers well-organized, first-class active vacations to some of the most exciting destinations in the world.

Whole Journeys
Europe, South America, Hawaii, Central America, India
877-745-4648
www.wholejourneys.com

Whole Journeys offers cultural walking adventures for travelers looking for an active, healthy travel experience with a small group of like-minded people. If you're looking to enrich your life by walking the "unbeaten path" in a small group, with authentic, comfortable accommodations and cuisine, extremely personal service, and a flexible itinerary, you'll love what Whole Journeys has to offer.

Clubs, Organizations, and Web Sites

American Volkssport Association (AVA)
Universal City, TX 78148
210-659-2112
Information line: 1-800-830-WALK
www.ava.org

The AVA offers noncompetitive walking events for everyone and is a network of over 500 clubs that organize more than 3,000 events per year in all 50 states.

North America Race Walk Foundation
PO Box 50312
Pasadena, CA 91115-0312
626-441-5459
members.aol.com/RWNARF/

NARF provides a wide variety of information. The Foundation specifically networks inquirers with racewalkers and racewalking clubs throughout the country. They have the latest information on shoes, technique, and training, as well as on current and past competitive times made by men and women of all ages. In addition, they have pamphlets on starting racewalking clubs and on judging procedures for those with these interests.

Racewalk
www.racewalk.com

The official racewalking home page of USATF provides all the information you need to start and improve your walking program and increase your awareness of other events in the walking community.

Walker Town USA
www.walkertownusa.com

The "home of competitive walkers willing to open their doors so that others may enjoy the sport." The site was developed so that walkers all over the world could have a single location to visit and be able to locate one of the many walking clubs available. Walking clubs from all over have sent in information, so that every level of walker (Competitive Racewalker, Non-Competitive Racewalker, Powerwalker, or Fitness Walker) can locate and learn more about them.

Foot Care

American Academy of Orthopaedic Surgeons (AAOS)
6300 North River Rd.
Rosemont, IL 60018-4262
Voice toll-free: 1-800-346-AAOS or 1-800-824-BONES
Voice: 847-823-7186
www.aaos.org

This resource serves as an advocate for improved patient care and informs the public about the science of orthopaedics. It also offers patient education, discussion groups, and a search vehicle to find orthopedic surgeons in your area.

American Podiatric Medical Association (APMA)
9312 Old Georgetown Rd.
Bethesda, MD 20814-1698
Voice toll-free: 1-800-FOOTCARE
Voice: 301-530-2752 or 301-571-9200
www.apma.org

The primary mission of the APMA is to advance the quality of foot care in the United States and to raise the awareness of the importance of foot health among the American public. They offer a variety of information on foot health, including foot facts and foot tips. They also list a series of helpful publications and educational resources, as well as a locator for a podiatrist near you.

Dr. Scholl's
www.drscholls.com

Besides having an online advice and care center, Dr. Scholl's also has an on-wheel Mobile Foot Care Center to deliver foot care advice, product samples, coupon booklets, and even a couple of foot massages to people all over the country. They sell many products ranging from inserts to cushions to heel cups and liners.

Footcare Express
2980 Aventura Blvd.
Aventura, FL 33180
877-687-3338
www.footcareexpress.com

Footcare Express carries the very latest in high-end foot care products that include, among other things, arch supports and insoles, custom-made orthotics, and various other foot care items. Footcare Express also carries various high-end performance, therapeutic, and comfort shoes.

Foot Levelers
518 Pocahontas Ave., N.E.
PO Box 12611
Roanoke, VA 24027-2611
1-800-777-4860
www.footlevelers.com

"Foot Levelers has created a line of custom-made, flexible orthotics to help feet properly support the body. We're always researching, designing, and producing quality custom-made orthotics which are scientifically designed for the individual's unique postural problems."

Spenco Medical Group
6301 Imperial Dr.
Waco, TX 76712
1-800-877-3626
www.spenco.com

Spenco is dedicated to delivering premium quality products that provide significant performance and enhancement benefits to both consumers and customers alike. They specialize in rubber-based insoles for added cushioning for the heel, arch, toes, and the entire foot.

Books and Magazines

Back Packer Magazine
33 East Minor St.
Emmaus, PA 18098
610-967-8296
www.backpacker.com

This site and magazine has a large list of walking, hiking, and backpacking locations found by state, city, and/or desired distance.

Walking Magazine
PO Box 5073
Harlan, IA 51593
1-800-829-5585
www.walkingmag.com

This is an easy-to-read reference for those looking for information on shoes, nutrition, strength, warming-up and stretching routines, event locations, walking inquiries, and more. You can subscribe to the magazine or just log on and read.

Outside Magazine
400 Market St.
Santa Fe, NM 87501
www.outsidemag.com

An informative magazine that offers news, features on adventure sports and wilderness destinations, and reviews of outdoor gear.

Fenton, Mark. *The 90-Day Fitness Walking Program.* 1995.

A daily walking program that helps strengthen the heart, burn fat, and improve fitness in 90 days, including information on how to choose the right shoes, warm up properly, utilize walking sticks and weights, and more.

Iknoian, Therese. *Fitness Walking.* Human Kinetics, 1995.

This book is an easy-to-read reference aimed toward the beginning, intermediate, and advanced walker looking to follow sample programs designed in four-week intervals.

Jacobson, Jake. *HealthWalk to Fitness.* HeartFit Books, 1999.

This book will teach you the proper techniques of healthwalking as well as sensible nutritional advice and some excellent stretching routines in an eight-week training program. Jacobson also offers a 14-day "Healthwalk Your Weight Off Program" for those of you who want to drop a couple pounds. The book is written for walkers of all fitness levels and ages.

Malkin, Mort. *Aerobic Walking: The Weight-Loss Exercise.* John Wiley & Sons, Inc., 1995.

This book features information on diet, footwear, safety, walking techniques, medical considerations, motivation, program design including distance, pace and quantity, and more. Somewhat on the technical side but very informative, Dr. Malkin teaches you how to walk down your weight, slow down the effects of aging, and walk toward a better, healthier you.

Mouland, Michael. *The Complete Idiot's Guide to Camping and Hiking.* Alpha Books, 1998.

This guide teaches ways to choose tents, sleeping bags, hiking boots, and more; learn what to pack—and what to leave behind; navigate trails with a compass and map; and how to avoid and handle emergency situations.

Rippe, Dr. James M., and Anne Ward. *Rockport Walking Program.* Prentice Hall Press, 1989.

This book involves a 30-day walking and nutritional program aimed at improving your health and fitness by lowering your cholesterol and body fat through healthy eating and walking. Dr. Rippe includes cookbook recommendations, a food diary, an exercise log, and recipes, as well as sample meal plans.

Smith, Kathy. *Walkfit for a Better Body.* Warner Books Inc., 1994.

Kathy's book is a compact yet informative resource on the why's, where's, and how to's of starting a walking program. She includes tips on walking through weight loss and pregnancy as well as suggestions for stretches and upper-body strengthening.

Other Resources

About.com

This is a very informative site that offers an abundance of information on and about anything and everything related to walking, including apparel, shoes, clubs and agencies, beginners' programs, injuries, and more.

InteliHealth
1-888-244-4636
www.intelihealth.com

A great healthy Web site that features information on an assortment of medical conditions such as diabetes, cancer, strokes, heart disease, and more. There are also links to fitness and sports medicine, as well as a medical conditions center and health-assessment page.

Video Fitness
PO Box 710221
Oak Hill, VA 20171-0221
www.videofitness.com

Anything and everything you want and need that has to do with video fitness, including a beginners' corner, reviews, a mentor program, and instructor index. This site offers videos on dance, walking, martial arts, body conditioning, and more.

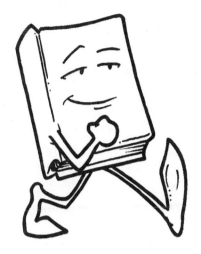

Walking Words

ACSM   The American College of Sports Medicine, considered the institution with the "gold standard" for exercise prescription and instruction.

active rest   The lower-intensity intervals between each high-intensity interval.

adhesions   The abnormal union of separate tissue surfaces by new fibrous tissue resulting from an inflammatory process.

Astroturf   A man-made, synthetic fiber, grass-like carpet structure with the associated backing fabric and shock-absorbing underpad or cushioning materials required for sports and recreational uses.

at training   Also known as anaerobic threshold training, refers to working at an intensity that is high enough where oxygen can no longer supply the need for energy. Energy, instead, is supplied through the anaerobic (without oxygen) system.

atherosclerosis   Literally "hardening of the arteries"; it is a cardiovascular disease that can lead to heart attacks and strokes.

atrophy   Comes from the Greek word *atrophos,* which means "ill-fed." It is the decrease in size or wasting away of a body part or tissue.

BMR   The basal metabolic rate is the energy expended by the body at rest to maintain normal bodily functions.

bunion   Also known as Hallux Valgus, a bunion is a condition in which the joint at the base of the big toe becomes malformed.

capillaries   Tiny blood vessels that transport and transfer nutrients and waste products to and from these tissues.

cardio   Refers to cardiovascular endurance, or the portion of your workout where you are pushing your heart and lungs for a continuous amount of time.

chondromalacia   The wearing away of the cartilage underneath the kneecap.

confidence   Having faith or belief that one will act in a right, proper, or effective way. Self-confidence is confidence in oneself and in one's powers and abilities.

continuous-duty   A treadmill's horsepower rating for steady, continual, 24-hour motor usage.

cortisol   A hormone found in the system after the body has endured high levels of stress. People who exercise too hard and too often without giving themselves adequate time to rest may have increased levels of cortisol in their systems.

Cross-training   Refers to incorporating more than one type of exercise into your weekly program.

dew point   The temperature at which a vapor begins to condense. Dew points are sometimes reported and/or used rather than relative humidity.

endorphins   Abbreviation of endogenous morphine, these brain chemicals are a special class of opiate-like substances released by the brain and pituitary gland that act as pain relievers in the body.

energy balance equation   Equation that states that to lose weight, you must consume fewer calories than you burn or, in reverse, you must burn more calories than you consume.

erector spinae   The muscles that run along your back and keep your spine erect.

fartlek   A Swedish word that translates as "speed play."

fibromyalgia   A condition of chronic muscle pain characterized by body aches, pain, sleep disturbances, fatigue, and anxiety, in combination with tenderness in 11 of 18 specific places on the body.

flexibility   The ability to move a joint through its full range of motion.

gait   The sequence of foot movements that defines the pattern in which a person walks.

gluteus maximus   Also known as the buttocks, the gluteus maximus are two of the largest and most powerful muscles in the body.

humidity   The amount of moisture in the air. The more vapor, the less evaporation of perspiration.

hyperglycemia   A condition in which too much glucose is in the bloodstream.

hypertension   The medical term for high blood pressure.

hypertrophy   Another word for increased muscle size or an enlargement of a muscle due to an increase in the size of the cells.

hypothalamus   The part of the brain that is resposible for the regulation of eating. It signals to our stomach when it is full and when it is not about 10 minutes after digestion has begun.

hypothermia   Heat loss or low body temperature.

insulin   A hormone secreted by the body that helps regulate the level, use, and transportation of sugar into and through the bloodstream and cells.

interval training   Involves repetitive sequences of high-intensity exercise bouts with low-intensity active recovery.

kyphotic   Refers to a forward curve of the head, shoulders, and pelvis as in the shape of a C.

lactic acid   The waste product left in your tissues during and after exercise, believed to be caused by inadequate oxygen in the muscle tissue during exercise.

major muscles   Refers to the larger, more active muscles, beginning with your legs and arms and ending with your stomach and back.

metabolic rate   Refers to the energy expended to maintain all physical and chemical changes occurring in the body.

microsystem   An area of the body that is a small representation of the whole body. It has been found through thousands of years of experience that the ears, hands, and feet are such areas.

motion-control shoes   The most rigid shoes. They are designed to be inflexible because they are meant to limit over-pronation. They are generally heavy but durable. Many are built upon a straight last with the denser material on the inside of the foot to help correct for pronation.

muscle endurance   The ability of the muscle to exert force continuously without fatigue.

muscle soreness   Also referred to as DOMS or Delayed Onset of Muscle Soreness. DOMS is thought to be a result of microscopic tearing of the muscle fibers. Swelling can occur in and around a muscle, which can also cause soreness hours later.

obesity   Defined as having a BMI of 30 or greater or a body fat composition of 30 percent or more.

over-pronation   The excessive inward roll of the foot so that the arch becomes completely flat.

over-supination   The excessive external rotation of the foot so that the arch is too high.

over-training   Physical and mental fatigue caused by working your body at a higher workload without giving it adequate time to rest, recover, and adapt.

overload   The principal that strength, endurance, and hypertrophy of a muscle will increase only when the muscle is overloaded by working it against loads that are above those normally encountered.

palpate   To examine through touch. When you determine pulse through palpation, it means you are measuring your heart rate by using your fingers.

pedorthics   The design, manufacture, modification, and fit of footwear to alleviate foot problems caused by disease, congenital defect, overuse, or injury.

peripheral vision   Relates to the outer part of the field of vision.

Pilates   A type of strength and stretching exercises originally designed for dancers.

plantar fasciitis   Also known as a heel spur, a condition causing pain localized over an area of the bottom of the foot near the heel.

plaque   The deposit of fatty substances, cholesterol, cellular waste products, calcium, and other substances in the inner lining of an artery.

plateau   A leveling off or evening out of change that is associated with, among other things, cardiovascular, strength, weight-loss, or flexibility programs.

polypropylene   A thermoplastic material exhibiting excellent cold flow, bi-axial strength, and yield elongation properties; it is similar to PVC but can be used in exposed applications because of it's excellent UV/weathering/ozone resistance.

power walking   A term often used to describe walking quickly and steadily for a good aerobic workout. A 13- to 15-minute mile is a good pace for power walking.

prime-mover muscles   Those muscles that are initiating and dominating a movement. For example, the prime mover in an arm curl would be the biceps, while the stabilizing muscles would be the shoulder and forearm muscles.

proactive   To act in anticipation of future problems, needs, or changes.

proprioception   Your body's ability to detect its movement through space.

relapse   The act or an instance of backsliding, worsening, or subsiding.

resting heart rate   A person's heart rate at rest.

ROM   Range of motion, which refers to the amount of motion allowed between two bony levers.

soft tissue   Your muscles and connective tissue and ligaments and tendons.

specificity   The principle that only those systems that are emphasized will adapt and change.

Spinning   An exercise class in which cyclists on special stationary, resistance-controlled bikes are led through an exercise routine by a certified Spinning instructor.

stabilizers   Those muscles in the front and back of your torso that support (stabilize) the spine. Your stomach and back are categorized as stabilizers.

subcutaneous fat   The lining of fat just underneath your skin.

supine   The position of your body when you are lying on your back; a term often used at the gym.

thermotherapy   Heat treatment.

trigger points   Areas of pain that appear throughout various parts of the body when a person is not well.

VLCDs   Very low-calorie diets that are usually no more than 800 calories and administered under the aid of proper medical care. They are not a recommended form of weight loss.

Volksmarch   A walking event. The name started in Germany, where these events were originally termed Volkswanderung—"volkswandering."

water weight   The number of pounds gained or lost by water retention and/or evaporation.

Index

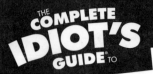